CHANGING HEALTHCARE ORGANISATIONS

ABOUT THE AUTHORS

DAVID COGHLAN is a member of the School of Business Studies, Trinity College, Dublin. He teaches and has published extensively in the areas of organisation development and action research. He participates actively in international networks in these areas and is the author of several books, including *The Dynamics of Organizational Levels* (with Nicholas Rashford in the Addison-Wesley OD series, 1994) and *Doing Action Research in Your Own Organization* (with Teresa Brannick, Sage, 2001).

EILISH MC AULIFFE is Director of the M.Sc. in Health Services Management at Trinity College Dublin. She teaches on organisational change. She has considerable experience of working with healthcare organisations. Eilish is the author of a number of books, including a co-authored book on organisational dynamics in international aid organisations, *Psychology of Aid* (with Stuart Carr and Mac MacLachlan, Routledge, 1998) and an edited book, *A Healthier Future? Managing Healthcare in Ireland* (with Laraine Joyce, IPA, 1998).

Changing Healthcare Organisations

David Coghlan
and
Eilish Mc Auliffe

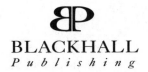

BLACKHALL
Publishing

This book was typeset by
ASHFIELD PRESS PUBLISHING SERVICES
for

BLACKHALL PUBLISHING
27 Carysfort Avenue
Blackrock
Co. Dublin
Ireland

e-mail: blackhall@eircom.net
www.blackhallpublishing.com

ISBN: 1 842180 52 5

A catalogue record for this book is available from the British Library.

£26·10

Printed in Ireland by
ColourBooks Ltd

Contents

Acknowledgements

We are grateful to colleagues and friends who provided us with support and valuable materials, Mary Casey, Brendan McCormack, Brendan MacPartlin and Don Warrick.

Our special thanks go to Warner Burke of Teachers' College, Columbia University, New York for permission to reproduce and develop the application of the Burke-Litwin model in chapter 4 to health systems, to Warren Bennis of the University of Southern California, for permission to use his change influence model in chapter 8, and to Rachel McKee of Grid International Inc. Austin, Texas who granted permission to reproduce the Grid material in chapter 9.

We are particularly grateful to the groups with which we have worked, who contributed to testing the constructs as they reflected on their own experience and contributed to change in the health system, particularly participants on the Organisation Development in Healthcare programme, successive cohorts of the Masters in Health Service Management at Trinity College and participants in the Masters in Nursing and Midwifery programmes in both Trinity College and UCD.

A special thanks is owed to Roger Nolan who took our handwritten diagrams and skillfully turned them into graphics. We acknowledge the invaluable help and support of the Blackhall editorial and production teams, especially Gerard O'Connor, Ruth Garvey and Susan Waine.

Foreword

Whole system change will be required in the Irish health system if we are to realise the goals in terms of health and social gain we have set out for the system over the period of implementation of the Health Strategy. Organisation change has deliberately been designated as one of the six frameworks for change.

Despite ongoing adjustment to management structures within many healthcare organisations, we have tended to accept the existing macro-structure as a relatively fixed point on the map, around which other aspects of change could be woven. This is set to change, following on the various reviews of structures, distribution of functions and governance arrangements within the system. The objective is to make the changes necessary to achieve better alignment between the challenges faced by the health system and the structures and processes through which people work.

As we move forward on this agenda of organisation change, we can only hope to succeed if we take full advantage of the experience of others and employ leading edge practice in shaping and carrying through the programme it entails.

This is the context in which *Changing Healthcare Organisations* will be closely read and valued by all who have an interest in the leadership and management of lasting change in the health system. In placing a welcome emphasis on the people issues around values, beliefs, culture and behaviour it offers a well-signposted route map through the challenging territory of managing large scale organisation change. The informative and reader-friendly treatment of key concepts and underlying theory, contextualised through real-life case studies, all set in a healthcare context, will make this a useful guide for experienced practitioners and novices alike.

Much of the development planned for the health system relies heavily on stronger commitment to teamwork and effective working of inter-disciplinary teams in a variety of care settings. The approaches to leadership and to managing change outlined will be found to be equally valid and informative for those contemplating change on this more local scale.

It is a hugely encouraging if sobering thought that, in any setting, most employees start out as well-motivated and enthusiastic contributors. Our continuous challenge as leaders and managers is to at least maintain and ideally grow that sense of positive contribution over each person's career cycle. This suggests a re-balancing of organisational priority towards human resource management in all of its aspects and an ongoing active concern for how the various attributes of structure help or hinder this process.

I welcome the publication of *Changing Healthcare Organisations* as a timely and valuable contribution to heightened awareness of this challenge and as a practical guide to all with an interest in addressing this challenge in the health system.

MICHAEL KELLY
Secretary General
Department of Health and Children

Preface

It is fast becoming trite to assert that new strategies are being demanded of managers at all levels of the Irish health system. Whether the managers are at health board CEO level, Assistant CEO level or at programme, project or ward level, none are exempt from the exigencies of change. Managers are continually working to deliver a quality service and to enable their organisational service delivery systems to be adaptable and flexible in order to deliver that quality service. Such work within health organisations involves a number of interconnected and interdependent issues. Examples of typical issues would include service planning and service delivery, HR systems that ensure an adequate supply of appropriately skilled staff and good relations between the organisation and its staff, effective communication, good team working, shared responsibilities to ensure integration between service delivery areas, effective information and communications technology, to name a few. Key to effective working of all this is a cadre of skilled professional managers and staff who can both enable the delivery of the service and build and maintain effective organisations and organisational units. Building and maintaining effective organisations will only be possible if such organisations are able to learn and change.

Readership

This book is aimed primarily at two groups of readers. The first group comprises of those who work in Irish health delivery organisations, whether in hospitals, health centres, health board administration, social services, in a senior, middle or front line management, or a service delivery role. We aim that this book will help you in your understanding and enactment of organisational change in your own organisation whatever your organisational role may be. The second group this book is aimed towards is the many people who are studying organisational change in the Irish health system at postgraduate and undergraduate levels in health service management and nursing programmes. This book provides an introduction to the core themes and issues in organisation development and change management in healthcare systems. The extensive references are aimed at providing further resources for your study.

Approach to Reading this Book

There are three main interlocking themes in this book. One is what we call "understanding organisations" where we discuss some key foundational themes, such as organisations as systems, how organisations function and, specifically, management and leadership, structure and strategy. The second theme is understanding the theory and practice of organisation development (OD as it commonly called) itself, and in particular large systems change, what resistance to change means, using consultants and other important topics. The third theme is the learning process itself, which we express in terms of action research or clinical inquiry.

In enacting an OD/action research approach to understanding your organisation and working at change, there are three broad strategies, which we are calling first, second and third-person research respectively. First-person research is about you, the individual person who is working in the health system or studying about it. This requires you to develop an inquiring approach to your own life and work. Hence, this book is adopting a "clinical inquiry" approach in which you are invited to attend to your own experience and what and how you are, so that you can learn in action. Clinical inquiry, along with other approaches to learning in action are described in more detail in chapter 3. Second-person research addresses your ability to inquire with others into issues of mutual concern and participate in teams, groups and action learning sets through the OD processes on which you work. Third-person research aims at creating a community of inquiry which is broader than those with whom you work directly and works at bringing the fruit of learning to the Irish healthcare system in general. At the end of each chapter, by means of "clinical inquiry" exercises and cases, we invite you to engage in first, second and third-person inquiry into your experience of yourself at work in your own organisation, into your experience of working with colleagues on change and into understanding how healthcare organisations can change.

Plan of the Book

The book is divided into three main parts. Part I Foundations lays out some of the organisational change issues in the Irish healthcare service, introduces organisation development and presents action research as the underlying philosophy of OD. Part II Understanding Organisations introduces two core frameworks for understanding the dynamics of organisational systems and therefore organisational change. Part III Organisation Development in Action focuses on the OD process itself and introduces a framework for large system change, discusses leadership, data gathering and evaluation, explores important issues such as resistance to change, using consultants and being an internal OD practitioner. At the end of each chapter there are case studies and reflective exercises to facilitate learning. The names of the organisations and people featured in the cases are fictional. The cases are aimed at stimulating personal reflection and class discussion, rather than as examples of good or bad practice.

PART I

FOUNDATIONS

CHAPTER I

The Case for Change

The contemporary world makes demands on the health service at each of its levels of complexity (Rashford and Coghlan, 1994). At the organisational level, the key task is the delivery of a quality health service to the public within government cost restraints. At the interdepartmental group level, the introduction and development of multi-disciplinary and inter-functional cooperation, organisational structures that emphasise lateral inter-service planning and service delivery are the requirement. At the team level the issues are the creation and maintenance of departmental team approaches to work and service delivery. At the individual level there are issues of performance and competencies, and through personal and professional development the individual employee is enabled to move from a bureaucratic mindset to a participative one sustained by an intrinsic motivation to provide the best possible care for the client or patient. Ultimately, an integrated service means that all four levels are working in harmony.

As if these issues in themselves are not challenging and difficult enough, there is an important complicating factor. Healthcare organisations are already in existence and have been for several decades. This means that there are structures, ways of working and shared attitudes already in existence and embedded in the collective psyche of the organisations and units. The task of management, therefore, is not only to build and maintain effective service delivery systems to meet the demands of today's world but to wean staff away from ways of thinking and working that belong to the past and that inhibit the forms of organisation and service delivery that are required to meet today's challenges. This was highlighted by Dixon and Baker (1996: vii) in their report: "Changing the culture of acceptance, deference and inertia is the most challenging aspect of the health strategy." All this means change. Managers themselves are not exempt from belonging to the mindsets of the past; they too need to work at changing themselves, while at the same time working at changing their organisations and units. Organisation development (OD) is the name given to planned change of the total system as a means of addressing the above-mentioned issues. It is not enough to focus on one or two particular issues, i.e. management development, team building, risk management or quality accreditation.

Figure 1.1 The Organisational Iceberg

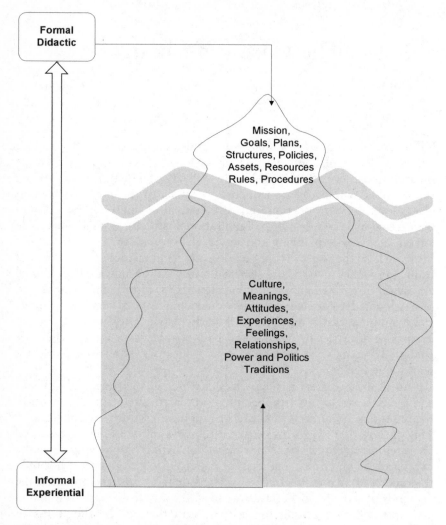

What is needed is a total system perspective that pays attention to a) each issue, b) how each issue is connected to each of the other issues and c) how a change in one creates a change in another.

In workshops and seminars on the subject of change in organisations, we frequently begin by asking the participants to list the words they associate with the notion of change. The subsequent list typically comprises such words as exciting, growth producing, improvement, energy, necessary and cooperation, and also words like threatening, anxiety, stress, fear, anger and force. What is clear is that change encompasses both experiences and that an experience of change can be both exciting and threatening at the same time. Accordingly, any attempt to understand and manage change must take this into account.

Organisations lead two lives. There is the public or formal life in which mission and goals are articulated, rules and procedures proscribed and lines of authority and responsibility defined. These elements can be found by studying the relevant documentation. There is also the hidden or informal life. This is the lived experience of an organisation, the area of perceptions, meanings, attitudes, feelings, experiences, traditions, informal relationships and interactions, power positions, methods of influence and so on. Only those who are on the inside, which is not readily available to outsiders, know this side of an organisation. These two organisational lives are frequently depicted as an iceberg – with the formal above the water and the informal hidden below the water line (Figure 1.1). As with icebergs, what is below and out of sight constitutes the larger portion. In the change process, both lives must be given attention. Members' experiences, their view of "how things really are" must be taken into consideration and worked with. It is better to work with the way things are rather than some model of how someone thinks they should be. Eminent social psychologist Kurt Lewin is credited with saying that one only understands an organisation when one tries to change it. This book pays particular attention to both organisational lives as they are manifested in healthcare organisations and in organisation development, and provides an important and useful approach to incorporating both in working to change and improve our health systems.

Case 1.1 Customer Care at St Mary's Hospital

St Mary's Hospital, a 500-bed acute hospital in a large urban area, decided it needed a customer care strategy. A multidisciplinary team of heads of disciplines and departments was established in order to develop this strategy. A key member of this team was the patient services manager, Tom Keane, as he was the person charged with sorting out any difficulties that arose with patients regarding their interaction with hospital staff.

At their first meeting the team were very enthusiastic and worked well together to produce a patients' charter that would form a basis for patients to judge the service they were receiving. All members of the team agreed to take the patients' charter to their own team or department to discuss it before their next meeting. At their second meeting some minor issues were raised regarding response times etc. and these were modified accordingly. All team members reported enthusiasm from staff on the patients' charter. The team spent this second meeting discussing how best to monitor adherence to the patients' charter in each area of the hospital. After much debate it was decided that a system of monitoring by the patient services manager

cont/d

might be perceived as too threatening and would likely give the impression that management did not trust staff to provide the quality of service set out in the patients' charter. It was therefore decided that the most acceptable way to monitor staff would be through patient/customer complaints. If there were a lot of complaints from patients, this would indicate that the charter was probably not being adhered to by staff. Three members of the team agreed to design a complaint form that would address the items set out in the patients' charter and would also allow patients to comment on other aspects of the service. This sub-group arrived at the third meeting with the newly designed complaint form and outlined how the process would work. Each ward/department/area in the hospital would have a box attached to a shelf and clearly labelled customer complaints. On the shelf beside each box a stack of complaint forms would be placed along with a pen attached to the box. At the end of each week Tom Keane would open the box, remove the forms, collate the information from them and give a brief report to the hospital management team on Monday morning at their regular weekly meeting.

The team adopted both the complaint form and the proposed process. Tom Keane discussed the team's work at the hospital's management team meeting the following Monday. It was subsequently approved by the management team, and the CEO, Martin O'Reilly, thanked the strategy team for its speedy response and good work. The boxes were manufactured and installed within the next two weeks and the system was launched by Martin O'Reilly, and declared operational two months after the first meeting of the strategy group.

At the first management team meeting following the introduction of this system, Tom Keane reported that only two forms (both of them very positive about the service) had been deposited in the boxes, although he had checked all 30 boxes that had been installed. The management team seemed surprised but it was suggested by the director of nursing, Ursula Hanson, that this was a positive sign and probably indicated that there was little to complain about as all staff were now adhering to the patients' charter. At the next management team meeting three forms had been collected, two very positive and complementary about the service and one extremely negative, complaining about waiting for three hours in outpatients and about the rudeness of staff. The complainant had also written on the end of the form that several other patients had also been kept waiting without any explanation for the delay. The management team began to wonder why there were not complaints from these other patients. Tom Keane was asked to investigate the matter further and report back to the next meeting.

Tom decided to ask around and get some opinions on how the system was working before trying to explore what had happened on the particular day the complainant had referred to. He asked a few of

cont/d

the ward managers if they felt the complaints system was working well on their wards. Two of them said it was working extremely well and patients seemed very happy with their care. Another said she assumed patients were happy because none of them had asked her for a complaint form to complete. From this, and subsequent conversations Tom had with nursing staff, it became apparent that the forms had been removed from the shelves for safe keeping and were held at the nursing station or reception area in each ward/department. Patients would need to request a form if they wanted to complete one and deposit it in the box.

It subsequently came to light through informal conversations with ward clerks that patients were not always given a form when they requested one, particularly if the staff were busy and the forms were not close at hand. Tom was left wondering if there was some other reason that staff wanted to hand out the forms themselves, particularly as each area in the hospital seemed to have adopted this strategy.

Questions
1. The complaints strategy clearly forms part of the formal organisation. Given what you have read, how would you describe the reaction to this strategy in the informal organisation?
2. How could the change process be adapted to ensure attention is given to the organisation's informal life?
3. What in your opinion needs to happen now to ensure that St Mary's Hospital adheres to its patients' charter?

ORGANISATION DEVELOPMENT AS AN APPROACH TO CHANGE

Organisation development is an approach to planned organisational change that has its own distinctive characteristics. These characteristics distinguish OD from a more general change management approach. What are these distinctive characteristics? We present four characteristics (French and Bell, 1999). (Figure 1.2)

Planned Change

There are different types of change. Some change is *reactive*: we are forced to react to some unforeseen event or crisis that must be dealt with. For example, if there is a major accident in an area, the Accident and Emergency department of the local hospital needs to react quickly by cancelling planned admissions to the hospital and deploying staff from other areas of the hospital to the Accident and Emergency department. Some change is *evolutionary*: it occurs in small increments over time and

Figure 1.2 Characteristics of Organisation Development

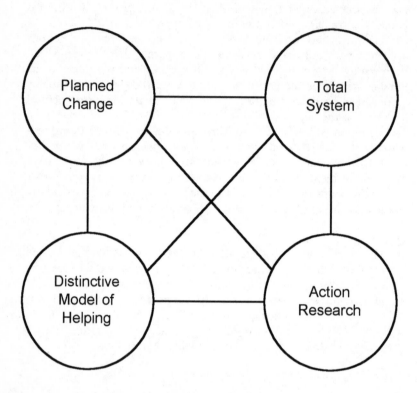

may not be particularly noticeable at any given point of time. An example of an evolutionary change is the gradual increase in day surgery over the past ten years, where improved technology and increased demand for services have played a role in gradually increasing the number and variety of surgical procedures offered on a day-case basis. Some change is *revolutionary*: a radical change is made quickly, for example the introduction of new nursing management structures and grades to the Irish health services. Another form of change is one where problems with a present situation are identified, alternatives are sought and selected, and a changed situation is deliberately created. A recent example of this type of change is the formation of the Eastern Regional Health Authority and the three area health boards to address the problem of poor integration of services for the population of the eastern region. This is referred to as *planned* change. When organisations, as complex social systems, attempt to initiate and manage planned change, they must acknowledge the complexity of the process and go about it in an organised manner. This is the subject of this book.

Total System

Organisation development as a process of planned change focuses on the total system. By "process" we mean *how* things are done and by "the total system" we mean not only the formal system of strategies, structures, authority, roles and procedures but also the informal system of relationships, networks, culture, history, attitudes and so on. The total system not only refers to all these elements individually but also to how they interact with one another and how they affect each other. A system can range in size from an individual ward or department, to a hospital, a health board or the total health system. Another important way in which organisations are systems is how the relationships individual employees have with the organisation and it with them is integrally related to how people participate in teams and groups, how these teams and groups relate to one another across structures, services, disciplines and geographical distances, and how individuals, teams, the interdepartmental groups contribute to the success of the organisation's delivery of its services.

Action Research

As the term suggests, action research is an approach to research that aims at both taking action and creating knowledge about that action. The outcomes are both an action and a research outcome, unlike traditional research approaches that aim at creating knowledge only. Action research works through a cyclical process of consciously and deliberately a) planning, b) taking action, c) evaluating the action, leading to further planning and so on. The second dimension of action research, taking action, is that it is participative, in that the members of the system participate actively in the cyclical process. The action research approach is powerful. It engages people as participants in seeking ideas, planning, taking actions, reviewing outcomes and learning what works and does not work, and why.

A Distinctive Helping Model

Organisation development is based on a set of values that can be expressed simply. The OD approach is to help organisation members to learn to solve their own problems and manage their own change so that they can learn how to continue to do so in the future. As change typically makes demands on people that require additional skills and resources, they need to access and utilise the kind of help that is most appropriate to their needs. Sometimes they seek out external professional expertise – someone who will give them relevant advice or information. At other times they seek a kind of help whereby they are enabled to learn themselves and the professional helper acts as the facilitator of their learning. It is this latter approach that is the hallmark of the OD approach.

The seminal works of psychologists Kurt Lewin, Carl Rogers and Edgar Schein have made significant contributions to the development of theories of how people learn and change. Some of the themes from their work are that people do not like to change unless they feel the need for it and value what the change will bring. People will find change difficult and will resist it more forcibly if they feel under threat. Accordingly, a central element in helping change take place is the reduction of threat and the creation of a sense of psychological security. Another element in change is that people change more easily when they feel they have a say in the change. We will return to these themes as we deal with particular elements of the change process.

To synthesise these characteristics, OD is about addressing planned change in an organisational system which itself is a complex reality of formal structural elements alongside the lived reality of how "things really are". Accordingly, it is important to keep a total system perspective, even when working with a particular part of it. What OD brings is a value-based approach that emphasises working in a collaborative and facilitative way with people to a) see how things are in the system, b) understand why it is the way it is, c) plan and enact appropriate actions to deal with the concerns arising from the view of the reality and d) evaluate those actions, learn from the experience in order to see how things are now and what actions might next be considered (Coghlan and Brannick, 2001).

OD as an approach to organisational change is particularly relevant to healthcare systems, not least because they are complex entities within which the knock-on effects of introducing change in one aspect of the system are all too obvious in other parts or sub-systems. The value-based approach that is inherent to OD is particularly suited to a service that is dependent on the staff in that system sharing the same set of values and the overriding aim of restoring people to full health. Health professionals by virtue of their education and training are familiar with the concepts of diagnosing problems and through consultation with colleagues, prescribing or planning a course of action to restore well-being to an individual. One could argue that the OD approach applied to organisations follows a similar process. A healthcare organisation can develop an illness or malaise and become stuck in a rut. It may need a commonly agreed diagnosis and prescription to overcome this malaise and break out of the rut, thus allowing the organisation and the people within it to develop and perform more effectively. Indeed, Cooklin (1999) and Coghlan (2002) argue that clinicians' professional clinical knowledge and their direct experience of how the organisation actually functions can be brought together as preunderstanding on which inquiry as to how to understand and treat organisations can be based.

Clinical Inquiry Exercise 1.1

Taking your own organisational system, in the blank iceberg (Figure 1.3)
1. Fill in the formal organisation.
2. Fill in the informal organisation.
3. Identify where there are inconsistencies between the formal and the informal.
4. Consider how the inconsistencies might be reconciled.
5. What might be done to achieve that reconciliation?

Figure 1.3 The Organisational Iceberg in Clinical Inquiry

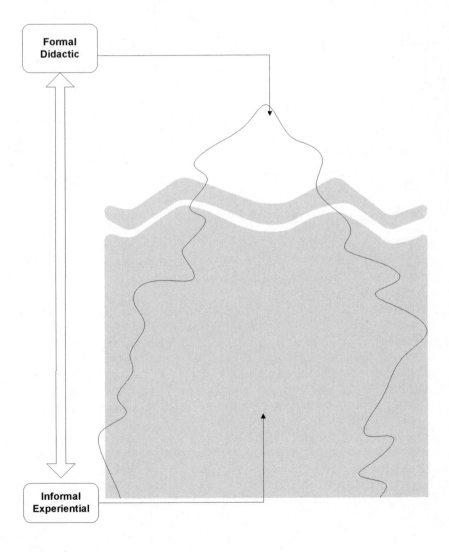

Clinical Inquiry Exercise 1.2

Re-read Customer Care at St Mary's Hospital (Case 1.1)
1. Taking a total system perspective, identify the key issues the strategy team should have considered in developing a plan for this change.
2. Design a process that you think will deal effectively with all the issues you have identified.

CHAPTER 2

Understanding Organisation Development

The approach we advocate for changing healthcare organisations is the organisation development approach. This differs in many respects from other approaches to planning, implementing and evaluating change in organisations. An important part of this difference is organisation development's attention to *process*, i.e. how change is implemented as distinct from *content*, i.e. what is actually changed. Many approaches focus primarily on content, whereas organisation development recognises the importance of both. This chapter, in explaining what organisation development is about and in distinguishing it from the other common approaches to change, highlights the centrality of attention to *process* as a key strategy in implementing successful and lasting change.

APPROACHES TO PLANNED CHANGE

In a classic article, Chin and Benne (1985) reviewed the literature on introducing planned change into human systems – such as social movements, education, psychotherapy – and summarised all the approaches into three groups of strategies: empirical-rational strategies, power-coercive strategies and normative re-educative strategies. Chin and Benne's work has been applied to health care systems, particularly nursing (Haffer, 1986; Cutliffe and Basser, 1997; Rimmer and Johnson, 1998).

Each group of strategies is based on different assumptions about the change process. *Empirical-rational* strategies are based on the assumption that the human person acts on the basis of rationality in line with self-interest in determining changes in behaviour. The change process, therefore, is one in which the information on which the change is based is studied so as to clarify its desirability and effectiveness. The change is adopted if it can be justified rationally through presentation of research data, argument and persuasion.

Under *power-coercive*, Chin and Benne emphasise the power of political and economic sanctions in the change process. In this approach change is brought about by manipulation of coalitions. This can be done by management exercising its power to enforce structural changes, or it can be done by generating mass support for change and using non-violent political means.

Normative re-educative is the name for the third group of strategies. This approach is based on assumptions which emphasise the developmental and social nature of the human person. Therefore, change processes typically focus on changes in attitudes, values and behaviours as well as knowledge. Changes such as these will necessarily involve a realignment of significant relationships and will pay attention to the forces which promote and impede change. Change involves "unlearning" old attitudes and behaviours and "relearning" new ones. For instance, people's fears and anxieties, their perceptions, the membership of groups, the norms and culture of those groups are significant forces in whether a change is accepted or resisted. Normative re-educative strategies for change focus on a system's abilities to solve its own problems. So there is an emphasis on experience-based learning and skills development so that members of the organisation can make the changes themselves in line with the issues which they identify as significant for their organisation.

When these different approaches to initiating and managing change in organisations are reviewed, it can be seen that some of the approaches and their subsequent strategies are based on different assumptions about how change takes place. Organisation development is an approach to planned organisational change which is grounded in normative re-educative assumptions and focuses on helping organisations manage their own change.

A prime example of a normative re-educative approach is Lewin's famous three stage change theory (Schein, 1980). Lewin found that for systems to change they must:

1. See the need for change (a stage which he called *unfreezing*).
2. Change from a present state to a future state (which he called *moving*).
3. Ensure the change survives and works (which he called *refreezing*).

In Lewin's theory, each stage is equally important. Unless the three stages occur change will not survive. Lewin's change theory has been the foundation of organisation development theory and practice for many generations for two reasons. First, many of the founders of organisation development were either directly influenced by Lewin himself or were influenced by his associates. Second, Lewin's theory exemplifies what organisation development is about. In organisation development theory and practice, issues of unfreezing, moving and refreezing are of equal importance. In an organisational change situation, it may be necessary to devote a great deal of time and energy to helping members of the organisation understand and appreciate the need for change. Not to do so may result in increased conflict and alienation and indeed the failure of the change process.

Thus in the development of the Health Strategy much attention was focused on gathering opinions and concerns (from users and providers) about the existing health system. This information painted the picture of why change was necessary. It may also be necessary to devote considerable attention to helping the change survive and work, so that the system does not revert to its former habits. Hence the need for a well-supported implementation plan. Given the limitations of the empirical-rational (that change only occurs when we have convincing information) and power-coercive (that those more powerful can force those less powerful to change) approaches to change, organisation development recognises that in normative re-educative approach culture, social systems, habits, resistance to change, attitudes and feelings are central to both understanding and managing the complexities of a change process.

We must acknowledge that Lewin's framework is under question in today's turbulent change times. Lewin's framework suggests that a) change is linear and b) a period of change is followed by periods of stability. We know that neither is true. Unfreezing, moving and refreezing can overlap. There is little stability to today's world so that the only constant is change itself. Many OD scholars find Lewin's notion of refreezing, meaning stabilisation, to be inapplicable to contemporary organisations. On the other hand, Weick and Quinn (1999) argue that episodic change follows Lewin's stages of unfreezing-moving-refreezing while continuous change follows a freeze-balance-unfreeze pattern. MacLachlan and Mc Auliffe (2003: 203) point out that an important feature of Lewin's theory is its explicit acknowledgement that stability reflects a dynamic of interacting forces, not simply a failure of something to happen. They point out the implications of this for development.

> Rural peasant communities in many developing countries are sustained through a way of life that may have changed little over hundreds of years. Yet this does not mean that such communities are stagnant. If instead they are seen as a "successful" balancing act, between opposing forces, then the would-be "developer" must approach "community development" with a new set of questions. Instead of asking "Why have these people not developed more?", a better approach may be to ask "Why has this situation continued to exist?" and "What forces are involved in maintaining the balance here?"

Although these authors are writing about working with communities in developing countries, the implications are equally valid when working with health systems in more developed countries. Lack of progress should not be dismissed, but explored in a way that provides information about potentially successful approaches to change.

Another useful construct with regard to laying some foundations for understanding organisation development is Kelman's (1969) distinction between three different responses to change initiatives. One may adopt a change through *compliance*, that is through the fear of sanction, i.e. "If I don't do it my manager may not support my application for promotion." Another approach is through *identification*, where change is adopted to identify with an individual or cause, i.e. "I'll do it because everyone else in my department seems to be in favour of it and I don't want to seem like the odd one out." The third form, *internalisation*, is that where change is adopted from a judgement of value that it is a good thing or the best alternative or so, i.e. "I'll do it because I really believe it will result in improved patient care." It is obvious that for a change to be sustained, a disposition of internalisation is more effective than compliance or identification.

WHAT IS ORGANISATION DEVELOPMENT?

Organisation development is an approach to planned organisational change. One of the earliest definitions was provided by Beckhard (1969: 9) a founder of OD:

> [A]n effort (1) planned, (2) organisation-wide, (3) managed from the top, to (4) increase organisation effectiveness and health through (5) planned interventions in the organisation's "processes" using behavioural-science knowledge.

French and Bell (1999: 26) in their widely-used, standard OD textbook provide a more developed definition.

> Organisation development is a long-term effort, led and supported by top management, to improve an organisation's visioning, empowerment, learning and problem-solving processes, through an ongoing, collaborative management of organisational culture – with special emphasis on the culture of intact work teams and other team configurations – utilizing the consultant-facilitator role and the use of theory and technology of applied behavioural science, including action research.

The above definitions provide something of the flavour of OD. The common elements in the many definitions focus on long-term organisational change, supported by top-management, using behavioural science in a manner that enables the organisation to learn about itself and develop change skills (Hanson and Lubin, 1995). OD emphasises employee participation in diagnosing problems and in finding and implementing solutions to those problems and evaluating the results. For within an OD approach, everyone in the organisation who is affected by the change should have the opportunity to contribute to the continuous-improvement process.

CHARACTERISTICS OF ORGANISATION DEVELOPMENT

The following characteristics mark the distinctiveness of organisation development as an approach to managing change. These characteristics distinguish OD from a more general change management approach (Worren et al. 1999; Farias and Johnson, 2000).

- OD is a process for building healthy, high performance organisations and improving and realising the full potential and self-renewing capabilities of organisations, groups and individuals. It is also an education-based strategy using a positive and constructive approach to successfully leading and managing change.

- OD is an interdisciplinary approach that draws primarily from the applied behavioural sciences (e.g. psychology, sociology) and uses understanding of business and the influence of technology on organisations.

- OD is values-driven and seeks to instil values and build cultures that bring out the best in organisations and people and to encourage open, straightforward, helpful, ethical and increasingly self-directing behaviour.

- OD is a facilitative process that helps others discover and find solutions to their own issues.

- OD relies on a systems perspective of organisations that considers all aspects of an organisation and its interrelated parts, i.e. focuses on the "big picture".

- OD is a data-driven, action research oriented approach that includes assessing reality and involving key stakeholders in evaluating results, exploring what is possible and planning further action.

- OD is a collaborative top-down, bottom-up process that recognises the importance of building the commitment and leadership of top-level decision makers and involving all stakeholders in the change process.

- OD focuses on both process (how things are done) and content (what is done) recognising the importance of both.

- OD is often guided and facilitated by professionally trained change agents, both external and internal.

- OD is committed to the transfer of knowledge and skills and to creating learning organisations where organisations and their members are continuously learning, sharing knowledge and improving the organisation.

• OD emphasises the importance of planned, lasting and sustained change, rather than the 'quick fix', while at the same time developing the organisation's ability to adapt to changing times.

It is important that we do not view organisations, and therefore organisation change also, in mechanical terms. A great deal of organisational language suggests that organisations can be changed like machines; "reengineering" is a good example of such use of language. Because organisation development is grounded in behavioural science it builds from the perspective of the people in the organisation. Accordingly, organisation change is fundamentally about conversation, where change happens because people are talking with each other about what is important and that conversations ultimately lead to psychological, behavioural and operational outcomes in the organisation. Change takes place through, and emerges out of conversation. As Pascale, Milleman and Gioja (2001: 203) put it, "Conversation is the source and soul of change". Hence the facilitation of conversation is a central dynamic of the work of organisation change.

CONTEXT FOR THE EMERGENCE OF OD

One of the contextual forces for the emergence of organisation development was the growing sense of the inadequacy of the bureaucratic model of organisation. Bennis (1969), in one of the first books on organisation development, presents the Burns and Stalker (1961) construct of mechanistic and organistic organisational systems. *Mechanistic systems* are those in which the emphasis is on authority-obedience relationships, strict division of labour, centralised decision-making and conflict resolution through suppression, arbitration and/or warfare. The central image in this description is that organisations are mechanisms which managers can work mechanically. Mechanistic systems are bureaucratic in their organisational form. They have a pyramid structure and are dominated by procedures for dealing with all contingencies related to work activity. *Organistic systems* are based on the image of the organisation as a living organism. In organistic systems, there is emphasis on interdependence and shared responsibility, mutual confidence and trust, wide sharing of responsibility and control, multi-group membership and responsibility and conflict resolution through bargaining or problem solving.

In Bennis' view, the mechanistic system is threatened by rapid and unexpected change, as the organisation's ability to respond to a changing world is lessened by its inflexibility and rigidity. Much of the change currently taking place in health systems involves the de-constructing of the old mechanistic bureaucratic-type organisations and the building of more organistic systems or healthcare organisations. In the past, the commonly held belief was that the paternalistic model of care with its emphasis on the treatment of specific diseases in passive patients could best be delivered in a bureaucratic, mechanistic structure – hence the existence of bureaucratic healthcare organisations divided along functional lines. More recently the emphasis has shifted towards a partnership approach to treating the whole person, whilst recognising that the patient has an important contribution to make in their recovery and that the interaction between clinician and patient influences this (Mc Auliffe, 1998). The preferred organisational model has become the organistic type. We see therefore a move from functional structures to client-centred or care group structures with much more emphasis on multi-disciplinary team work.

Another of the seminal organisation development writers, Argyris (1960) approached the mechanistic organisation from another perspective. Argyris contrasts the psychology of individual development with the impact formal bureaucratic organisations have on their individuals members. He puts forward a number of propositions which illustrate how the formal organisation, in its attempts to optimise its own efforts, actually negate the developmental thrust of individuals. Individuals tend to develop from a state of passivity as infants to a state of increasing activity as adults. They move from dependence on others to relative independence and inter-dependence. They move from having a few ways of behaving to being capable of behaving in many different ways. They move from having a short-term perspective to a much longer-term perspective. They develop a sense of self-awareness and self-reflection. They develop an ability to set personal goals and have values. Bureaucratic organisations, by adopting a short-term perspective, foster dependency and expect their employees to adopt a passive, dependent and subordinate stance (so also patients of bureaucratic healthcare organisations). Individuals are given minimal control over their work. They are expected to utilise a few skin-surface skills. The effect, in Argyris' view, is that bureaucratic organisations keep their employees immature.

In a similar vein, McGregor (1960) found that managers could be organised into two groups, operating from different sets of assumptions. One set of assumptions, which he called Theory X, operates under the assumptions that the human person does not like work and will avoid it if possible. Accordingly, managers must behave as if individuals cannot be trusted and must exercise control to ensure the work is done. McGregor found that the managers who worked from such assumptions created a self-fulfilling prophecy; they created workers who could not be trusted and who required close supervision. The second set of assumptions, which McGregor called Theory Y, assumes that the individual does not have an antipathy to work and so will, under the right conditions, accept responsibility, seek creative solutions to problems and can develop and mature.

There are many other developments in understanding the nature of people in organisations which had a major impact on the emergence of organisation development in the late 1950s, through the 1960s and on into the twenty-first century (Burke, 1994; French and Bell, 1999). Of course, organisation development has not stood still and is constantly interacting by influencing and being influenced by developments in contemporary organisational and management theory and practice (Burke, 2002).

One important example of a contemporary development in organisational and management theory and practice is the focus on organisational learning and dialogue (Argyris and Schon, 1996). In an age of increasing globalisation and technological advances it is becoming critical that organisations develop the practice and skills of learning.

Organisational learning refers to how organisations as systems learn, rather than how its individuals learn. Individual learning does not necessarily transfer to organisational learning. Senge's (1990) distinction between "generative" and "adaptive" learning is a distinction between the capacity for an organisation to reinvent itself, re-examine and evolve its assumptions and test them against new realities (generative learning), not merely to improve its capacity to adapt efficiently (adaptive learning).

As learning is a social process that occurs best in a group setting where the group is engaged in pursuit of a common and relevant task, the ability to engage in dialogue is central to organisational learning. Dialogue involves listening to one another and exploring meanings and assumptions to reach common understanding. A number of recent writings have emphasised the importance of dialogue in increasing understanding amongst health professionals and improving health systems (Plochg and Klazinga, 2002; Tremblay, 2002). Such dialogue is at the core of contemporary emphases on partnership between employers and employees, and so OD accommodates the conversation which takes place within an industrial relations framework (Shirom, 1983).

Another contemporary development is the perspective of organisations as complex adaptive systems. This view comes from biology, quantum physics and chaos theory, particularly theories of self-organisation, non-equilibrium, complementarity and "butterfly effect" where minute fluctuations can produce large-scale changes (Wheatley, 1999; Stacey, 2001). As Burke (2002) points out, organisations are living systems with patterns of relationships that determine the organisation's characteristics, with cultures that require deep change to alter, and cognitive processes of selectivity where they respond to some things and not to others. The thrust of these approaches is to argue that mechanical systems theory is not sufficient to understand organisations in their complex environments and that the life sciences have much to teach us about the characteristics of living systems. The corollary of these approaches is to play down approaches to change which attempt to control, as in top down strategic planning approaches, but rather to create the conditions whereby learning happens and change emerges through patterns of interaction. In these approaches the dominant image is not the military one of strategy, operations and tactics; rather it is the jazz group in which individuals self-organise and come together through creativity, differences and energy to form a whole.

THE EMERGENCE OF ORGANISATION DEVELOPMENT

Organisation development does not comprise a single theory and so its origins lie in many different strands of applied behavioural science – individual psychology, group dynamics, leadership, organisation theory, human resource management and elements from sociology and anthropology. In some respects organisation development builds on all the major developments of organisation theory and the interface of organisations with the people who work in them. Some of the experiments and research which are more directly related to the emergence of organisation development as a distinctive approach to managing planned change are:

1. The work of Kurt Lewin on re-education, participative change, field theory, the stages of change, action research and his seminal work on group dynamics, and in particular the emergence of sensitivity training.
2. The work of Eric Trist and his associates in the Tavistock Institute in the UK on coal mining in Durham which led to an understanding of how technology and people are interdependent and how organisations are socio-technical systems.
3. The client-centred approach to helping individuals make their own personal change pioneered by Carl Rogers.
4. The approaches to surveying organisations developed by Likert and his colleagues in Michigan.

Much of the development of OD came out of Lewin's discovery that attention to "here-and-now" processes in a group provides a powerful vehicle for learning about groups. This insight was formalised in the T-group (T stands for training), which is an unstructured group led by a trainer who works in a non-directive manner. T-groups were organised by the National Training Laboratories (later the NTL Institute), which was founded by Lewin's associates. NTL and T-groups are the most significant origin of organisation development because (a) the philosophy of the T-group, whereby the trainer works in a non-directive manner and learning takes place out of what is happening in the group (a paradigm of action research) and (b) the pioneers and significant developers of organisation development were T-group trainers in the NTL Institute (Golembiewski, 1989; French and Bell, 1999). It was when the T-group was being applied to working teams that the focus and the term "organisation development" emerged. In Britain, the Tavistock Institute developed its own form of the T-group in the Tavistock Conference and through its work on socio-technical systems paralleled organisation development.

The early approaches placed a great deal of emphasis on individual and group development. The task-focused nature of working teams in organisations and the hierarchical relationships within an organisation's structure challenged the T-group trainers to redefine their work beyond the personal learning in an egalitarian setting. The experiential learning dynamic of the T-group was now being applied to larger, more complex systems. This experiential learning, or action research as it was called by Lewin, was based on two assumptions which are the cornerstones of OD. One is that involving the clients or learners in their own learning, not only produces better learning but more valid data about how the system really works. The other is that one only understands a system when one tries to change it, as changing human systems often involves variables which cannot be controlled by traditional research methods. Accordingly, action research and its developments in action science and clinical enquiry evolved a science of practice (Greenwood and Levin, 1998). A central element of the OD approach, therefore, is an experiential approach which goes with the story as it evolves, rather than imposing defined programmes.

Weisbord (1987) traces an evolution of a theory of practice in the development of organisational change. In the early 1900s experts solved problems. In the 1950s everybody solved problems. In the mid-1960s experts improved whole systems and now as we move beyond 2000 everybody improves whole systems. It is in this regard that the normative re-educative philosophy of organisation development is pertinent. Organisation development practitioners work in a facilitative rather than an expert role. While OD practitioners have expertise in the fields of organisational and management theory, group dynamics, organisational psychology, change theory and so on, they use their expertise to help members of the organisation identify and solve their own problems. This approach contrasts with the more prescriptive expert-based approaches in which experts diagnose the problem and prescribe solutions which the organisation then implements.

How Does OD Differ from other Common Change Approaches?

Organisation development frequently draws on processes such as management development, training, total quality (TQM), action learning, teambuilding and many other organisational interventions.

- *Training* is an activity in which many organisations invest considerable resources. What can typically happen is that the focus is on the individual and the organisation does not change. Organisational structures, culture and processes may present obstacles to the newly trained individual as he/she tries to change his/her way of working. While training could be part of OD, the OD approach would work at integrating training into planned organisational change.
- *Management development* is really "manager development" and its purpose is to upscale the skills, capabilities and capacity of managers. These do not necessarily change the organisation unless they are linked to other elements of how the organisation works and what changes are planned. Managers' performance is not only influenced by managers' skills and capabilities but will also be strongly influenced by the reward system, the culture, etc.
- *Total Quality Management* is a total package approach to organisational change based on the methodology of continuous improvement. It is a task-focused approach that tries to enforce a uniform change across an organisation, which may not fit all parts.
- *Business Process Re-engineering* claims to be a radical approach to organisational change and builds on OD in the sense that it encourages managers to re-think what they do and how they do it in order to achieve greater efficiency and effectiveness. It differs from OD in that it tends to focus on short-term outcomes and often ignores the difficult concepts of power, politics and culture.
- *Teambuilding* typically means developing team leaders. Developing team leaders may not have its desired outcomes unless staff are helped to work as team members. Another pitfall is that a focus on teams may be undermined by a focus on the individual in the reward or promotion system. If rewards are based on individual performance, this may create a tendency for team members to compete with rather than cooperate with each other.
- *Performance management* is a system that aims to improve organisational performance by improving individuals' performance. This is achieved by setting goals and targets and measuring progress on the achievement of these goals. Performance is measured according to a pre-determined set of performance indicators. This can create difficulties as performance tends to improve in the areas for which indicators have been set, but this may have a knock-on negative effect on performance in other areas. Such a system can also create difficulties for collaborative working if rewards are based on individuals' performance, as is usually the case.

- *Action Learning* is an approach to the development of people in organisations which uses the *task* as the vehicle for learning. The learning process is based on a cycle of planning, action, reflection and evaluation. Participants work in teams or learning sets on real problems. The problems for the most part tend to be an individual's problems or a team's problems but rarely the organisational problems. As an approach it therefore has limited ability to impact on the total organisation.

What is important to note is that these interventions of themselves are not OD because they do not necessarily focus on the whole system. The overall point is that OD is system-oriented, based on the premise that organisations are complex and held together by interconnected and interdependent elements. A change in one can have a knock on effect on other elements (whether intended or unintended). While an OD approach may utilise management development, training and teambuilding, these of themselves are not OD as they don't have a total system perspective.

OD is likely to be used successfully when:

- There is a perceived need for change in the organisation.
- Senior managers are willing to commit themselves to long-term improvement.
- Senior managers are willing to involve members of the organisation in problem-finding and solution-generating activities.
- There is a core of trust and cooperation existing in the organisation.

OD is unlikely to succeed where management rules by fear and coercion, where there is no commitment to long-term change, where management has a preoccupation with the short-term fix to give the illusion of change and where there is deeply rooted political conflict and very low trust. OD is not the only alternative. In situations of crisis, where an organisation is facing extinction in the short term, drastic change is called for and so coercive approaches may be appropriate (Dunphy and Stace, 1990). In other situations organisational change may be brought about through planned and formal negotiation procedures.

It may appear that OD is actually good management practice. While a lot of OD techniques have been adopted by general management and are in everyday use, OD has retained its identity because it focuses on providing a service of helping organisations change.

ORGANISATION DEVELOPMENT IN HEALTHCARE SYSTEMS

The literature on OD in healthcare systems is sparse. In the US traditional applications of OD typically focus on hospitals (Margulies and Adams, 1982; Boss, 1989), and then more specifically on how OD can help the growing focus on quality and service (Freeman and Penrod, 1993; White, 1999). In the UK, there have been numerous OD interventions in the healthcare setting, but for the most part they have been focused on small group work, or OD interventions with sub-systems within the total system. During the 1980s there was strong interest in trying to create cultural change in organisations and the NHS did adopt some OD approaches in trying to create such change (Harrison and Robertson, 1985; Iles and Sutherland, 2001). For the most part, cultural change initiatives in healthcare met with limited success. Also an impatience with the length of time required to achieve cultural change in the context of a rapidly changing external environment, meant that more rapid approaches to the improvement of organisational effectiveness were advocated in the early 1990s (Buchanan, 1997). The rising popularity of business process re-engineering meant that consultants and researchers adopted this approach to analysing the ever more complex environment of acute hospitals. This reflected Beer, Eisenstat, and Spector's (1990) "task aligned" approach to change. They were critical of the "programmatic change" which is typical of most culture change programmes.

Buchanan, attempting to re-engineer an operating theatre, identified several problems with the approach including the difficulties of taking account of the different political agendas of the professions involved and the lack of precision in the approach allowing scope for political manoeuvring. He noted that BPR appears "insensitive to organisational history, context and politics, and as such sits outside the mainstream of organisation development theory and intervention where contextual sensitivity is generally regarded as a prerequisite for effective change" (1997: 69). Bate (2000a) describes a case study of a large-scale change programme within an NHS hospital using a socio-technical systems approach. The hospital which was moving to a new site struggled to transform itself from a rigid and divided hierarchy to a more flexible and collaborative "networked community". Bate highlights that the significant aspect of this particular case was that the process was "home grown – jointly designed and inclusive (an action research approach was employed), collaborative rather than coercive, and without preconception about specific final outcomes" (2000a: 509).

In Ireland little has been published on OD interventions applied to healthcare settings. However, the Irish health services, having focused traditionally on changing structures and developing mission statements and strategy to create improvements in organisations, are slowly beginning to realise that *process* may deserve more attention in the change agenda (Mc Auliffe, Coghlan and Pathe, 2002; Coghlan, Mc Auliffe and Pathe, 2002–3). This is exemplified by the approach taken in developing the 2001 Health Strategy, *Quality and Fairness: A Health System for You.* Extract 1 outlines the rationale for this approach and places strong emphasis on participation and consultation.

Extract 1 Approach to Development of the Strategy

DEVELOPMENT OF A NEW STRATEGY

Guiding Principles and Themes

The guiding principles underpinning the new Strategy are likely to emphasise a more people-centred/consumer oriented system, an analysis of cross-sectoral issues affecting health status and the development of integrated sets of quality services, accessed on the basis of need. There will also be strong focus on equity.

In addition to the agendas for service and professional development referred to above, key themes of the new Strategy are expected to include health futures, health promotion/population health, quality, information systems and e-health, delivery systems including human resource issues, funding and eligibility.

Approach

A participative approach and intensive consultation process is seen as crucial to the process of developing the new Strategy. Lead responsibility for production of the Strategy has been assigned to a Steering Group chaired by the Secretary General, Department of Health and Children (DOHC), and comprising the Department's Management Advisory Committee and a number of health board/Authority Chief Executive Officers. A Project Team has been established to produce the Strategy document under the overall leadership of the Steering Group. It includes representatives of the Department of Health and Children and of the health boards/Authority.

Gaining an understanding of the difficulties ordinary people face in achieving a better health status is essential to planning improvements. This underlines the need for a comprehensive consultation process. Accordingly, a broad ranging consultation process with the public, service users and providers and key stakeholders has been initiated. A National Health Strategy Consultative Forum, representative of key

cont/d

stakeholders in the health services, including health professionals, management and consumers...has been established to provide advice to the Steering Group...meetings of focused sub-groups of the Consultative Forum looking at key themes will take place over the next couple of months. It is hoped to hold the first plenary meeting of the Consultation Forum on...

In addition to the Consultative Forum, members of the general public and other interested parties will be consulted in a number of ways including a national advertisement inviting submissions and local level consultation.

In recognition of the cross-sectoral issues impacting on health, an Inter-Departmental Group is also planned to promote cross-departmental linkages. The Departments of Finance; Environment and Local Government; Education and Science; Enterprise, Trade and Employment; and Social, Community and Family Affairs will be invited to participate in this.

Source: http://www.doh.ie/hstrat/prephs.html

The shift that has resulted in a much stronger emphasis on process has been driven partly by a greater concern for employees (in the recent labour shortage) and also by the increasing complexity that has been created as a result of numerous structural changes. It is also noteworthy that the Department of Health and Children have extended the consultation process beyond the traditional boundaries of the health system and invited members of the public to participate as evidenced in Extract 2, which also appeared as a national advertisement.

Extract 2 Request for Submissions from the Public

HELP US PLAN THE HEALTH SERVICE YOU NEED

The Minister for Health and Children, Micheál Martin T.D., his Department and the Health Boards are working on a major new plan "Health Strategy 2001". The purpose of this Strategy is to develop health and personal social services over the next 5–7 years to meet your health needs and the needs of your family.

This is an opportunity for change. You have a real opportunity to help shape the future and decide priorities. We want to hear from members of the public, from organisations involved directly with health services, and from any group or organisation with a view about how we can best promote health and well being.

You can give your views in a number of ways and we have a

cont/d

consultation pack to help you. You can request a copy of the consultation pack "Your Views about Health" by writing to:

"Your Views about Health" , Department of Health and Children, Second Floor, Hawkins House, FREEPOST, Dublin 2 (no postage stamp is needed).

Or you can request the consultation pack in any of the following ways:

By Phone: Lo Call 1890 635459
By E-mail to: healthstrategy2001@health.irlgov.ie
By Fax: (01) 6354566

The consultation pack is available in Irish, and in Braille or on audio tape. You can request these by telephoning us at Lo-Call 1890 635459.

Source: http://www.doh.ie/hstrat/prephs.html

This advertisement is interesting in its attempts to include all those who might have a view about healthcare and in its attempts to make it as easy as possible for individuals to contribute their views. It differs substantially from traditional approaches to developing strategy which were much more "top down" and "expert led".

The multidisciplinary team approach has become an important concept in healthcare and there is recognition of the need for team building and process focused intervention. Also there is a greater emphasis on empowering staff, particularly nursing staff, to fulfil the increasing demands of their roles. The most popular OD interventions in the Irish health system have been team-building approaches, action learning groups and mentoring. The focus has been very much at the individual and group level. However, a number of organisations have begun to take a more systems-wide approach to OD. One organisation has developed an action learning programme for all middle management in the organisation and plans to extend this to other levels of management. Another has introduced an organisation-wide change programme using internal change agents to work on a number of prioritised change initiatives throughout the organisation. Yet another has taken a project management approach to introducing change, training a large number of staff in the techniques of project management and applying this model to all new initiatives or service developments throughout the organisation. Each of these organisations have built-in reflection and feedback loops as part of the process of change and whilst they may not be OD interventions in the purest form they each incorporate elements of the OD tradition.

CONCLUSIONS

In conclusion, organisation development addresses issues of how social systems change. Its theory base draws on those elements in the social sciences which have addressed how people function in systems and how systems change. In its normative re-educative philosophy OD attends to issues of internalisation, acknowledging the limitations of compliance and identification, and provides normative perspectives on how internalised change can be productive.

OD's focus on action research – the process of reflecting on experience – can enable the health system enquire into its experience by creating and testing assumptions and hypotheses in order to learn from experience. The health system as a community of enquiry can engage in its own cycles of enquiry, hypothesis formulation, testing, implementation and reflection on its experience in the contemporary world.

In this chapter we have introduced the notion of organisation development by defining it, describing its characteristics and illustrating how it emerged to deal with the limitations of mechanistic mentalities of organisations. We have built organisation development around the core construct of the normative re-educative approach to change which emphasises the centrality of the re-educative process, social relationships, culture and tradition, and the necessity of helping members of an organisation develop their own change management skills through dialogue.

Case 2.1 Integrating Cancer Services

The Northern health board is attempting to develop its cancer services in accordance with the National Cancer Strategy which calls for the development of regional oncology centres. The health board currently has cancer services on two sites. St Patrick's Hospital in Newcastle, at one end of the board's geographical area, has developed an expertise in breast surgery and also offers chemotherapy and some limited radiotherapy services. The breast cancer team includes a surgeon, a radiologist and three specialist oncology nurses. St Anne's, located 60 kilometres miles away in the town of Ballingar, at the opposite end of the catchment area, has a dermatologist with a special interest in skin cancers and an endocrinologist who has gained considerable experience (whilst working in the US) in the treatment of thyroid cancer. There are also two oncology nurses in the hospital. The consultants' ambition is to build a specialist oncology unit in St Anne's. The view of the health board and the CEO is that oncology services should all be located in Newcastle as it has a population of 200,000 whereas Ballingar's population is only 85,000.

cont/d

Although the consultants in both hospitals are prepared to work together to provide a comprehensive oncology service for the region, they fail to see the advantage of having it all on one site. In fact they believe that this is just a devious plot concocted by management to cut costs, and that it has nothing to do with providing the best service. The consultants counter all the arguments about the requirement of specified minimum throughput of patients necessary to maintain existing expertise and train new staff by stating that they are more than willing to work with their colleagues on the other site.

The situation is further complicated by the fact that there have already been two public demonstrations in Ballingar, one by several women's groups in the area arguing for the extension of the breast cancer services in Newcastle to Ballingar as the distance is too far for women receiving chemotherapy, particularly those who have young children and limited support networks. They argue that many of the women in receipt of services are not native to Ballingar but have moved there so their husbands could work in the local computer technology plant. The second demonstration which was attended by more than 800 people was to demand the development of specialist services for skin cancer, on the basis that this is the most common form of cancer and specialists in this area should be given the funding and support to develop services. Following this demonstration a rumour was circulated amongst the management of St Anne's that one of their consultants had orchestrated this demonstration, although no proof of this has surfaced. The health board has as yet made no response to either of these demonstrations.

Questions

1. In your opinion would an OD approach be appropriate to resolving this situation?
2. What are the factors that might mitigate against such an approach?
3. What factors are present that would lend support to an OD approach?
4. Which of these approaches do you think is likely to be most successful in bringing about change in this situation, and why?
   a) Empirical-rational
   b) Power-coercive
   c) Normative re-educative

Clinical Inquiry Exercise 2.1

1. Think of a change that has recently taken place in your own organisation.
2. Identify the factors present in the situation that might have contributed to a successful outcome if an OD approach had been adopted to bring about the change.
3. Identify the factors that would have made it difficult for an OD approach to succeed in the situation.

CHAPTER 3

Organisation Development and Action Research

Shani and Pasmore (1985: 439) provide a definition of action research that echoes our description of the theory and practice of organisation development in the previous chapter.

> Action research may be defined as an emergent inquiry process in which applied behavioural science knowledge is integrated with existing organisational knowledge and applied to solve real organisational problems. It is simultaneously concerned with bringing about change in organisations, in developing self-help competencies in organisational members and in adding to scientific knowledge. Finally it is an evolving process that is undertaken in a spirit of collaboration and co-inquiry.

The elements of action research, from this definition are clearly:

1. Taking a picture of the system relative to some identified issues.
2. Working with other members of the system as to what the data mean (a sort of "shared diagnosis").
3. Deciding what needs to be worked on in order to change the system in the desired direction.
4. Making planned interventions in the system on the basis of the planned action to achieve those desired changes.
5. Evaluating both intended and unintended outcomes and taking another picture of the system to see what needs to be done next, and so the cycle is repeated.

It is easy to see how these steps are similar to the steps OD practitioners use (Cunningham, 1993). Indeed, action research and OD are intimately intertwined, both theoretically and through the work of those scholar-practitioners who have shaped the development of both approaches.

Action research developed from the work of Kurt Lewin and his colleagues, and the colleagues with whom they in turn worked, who established a tradition of scholar-practitioners in group dynamics and social psychology. After Lewin's death, action research became integral to the growth of the theory and practice of organisation development. Argyris, Putnam and Smith (1985: 7–8) summarise Lewin's concept of action research.

1. It involves change experiments on real issues in social systems. It focuses on a particular issue and seeks to provide assistance to the client system.
2. It, like social management more generally, involves iterative cycles of identifying a problem, planning, acting and evaluating.
3. The intended change in an action research project typically involves re-education, a term that refers to changing patterns of thinking and action that are presently well-established in individuals and groups. Effective re-education depends on participation by clients in diagnosis, fact-finding and free choice to engage in new kinds of action.
4. It challenges the status quo from a participative perspective, which is congruent with the requirements of effective re-education.
5. It is intended to contribute simultaneously to basic knowledge in social science and to social action in everyday life. High standards for developing theory and empirically testing propositions organised by theory are not be to be sacrificed nor the relation to practice lost.

Figure 3.1 The Action Research Cycle

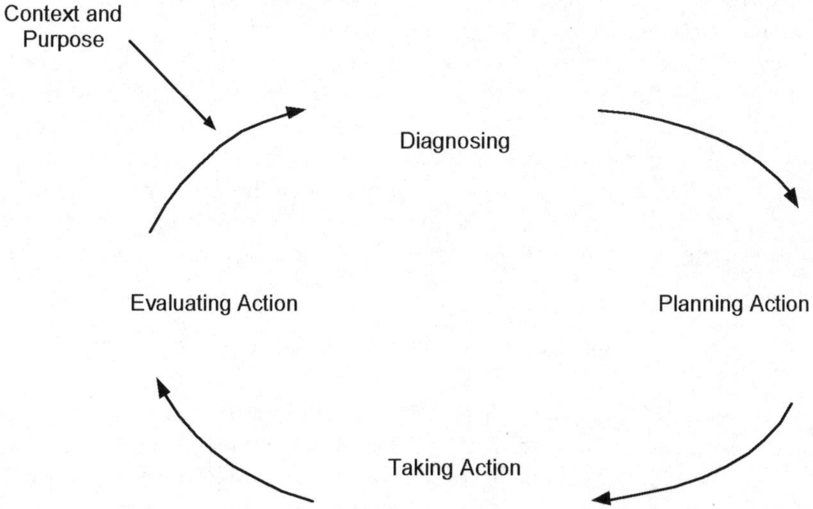

Source: *Doing Action Research in Your Own Organization*, David Coghlan and Teresa Brannick, Sage 2001: 17. Reproduced with permission.

What is distinctive about action research and OD is that both follow a cyclical process of consciously and deliberately a) diagnosing the situation, b) planning action, c) taking action, d) evaluating the action, leading to further diagnosing, planning and so on (Figure 3.1). The second dimension is that both approaches are participative, in that the members of the system participate actively in the cyclical process. The action research approach is powerful. It engages people as participants in seeking ideas, planning, taking action, reviewing outcomes and learning what works and does not work, and why. These are in stark contrast with programmed approaches that mandate following pre-designed steps and which tend not to be open to alteration. These approaches are based on the assumption that the system should adopt the whole package as designed. Action research and OD, on the other hand, are based on assumptions that each system is unique and that a change process has to be designed with that uniqueness in mind and adapted in the light of experience and learning.

Action research is well-established in healthcare organisations (Towell and Harries, 1978; Hart and Bond, 1995; Bate, 2000a; Morton-Cooper, 2000; Morrison and Lilford, 2001; Waterman, Tillen, Dickson and de Koning, 2001; Winter and Munn-Giddings, 2001). Journals such as the *Journal of Advanced Nursing* and the *Journal of Clinical Nursing* regularly feature explorations of its value and use action research in nursing (Webb, 1989; McCaugherty, 1991; Holter and Schwartz-Barcott, 1993; Rolfe, 1996; Coghlan and Casey, 2001). Examples of action research in the clinical area illustrate interventions to improve: pain management (Simons, 2002), stroke care (Gibbon and Little, 1995), palliative care (Cooper and Hewison, 2002), breast cancer care (Lauri and Sainio, 1998), and psychiatric and emergency services (Heslop, Elsom and Parker, 2000). Examples of action research in the organisational and operational areas include: care plan planning and audit (McElroy, Corben and McLeish, 1995; Webb and Pontin, 1997), continuous quality improvement (Potter, Morgan and Thompson, 1994), clinical teaching (Hyrkas, 1997), introducing clinical practice facilitators (Kelly and Simpson, 2001) and health visiting parenting programme (Kilgour and Fleming, 2000).

APPROACHES TO ACTION RESEARCH

Action research has developed to become a family of approaches, each with its own particular emphasis and yet all following the core tenets of reflecting on experience and participation (Greenwood and Levin, 1998; Reason, 2001). Examples of particular approaches within the family of action research are clinical inquiry, appreciative inquiry, reflective practice, action learning and cooperative inquiry. We now provide an overview of each in turn.

Clinical Inquiry

The distinguished organisational psychologist Edgar Schein (1987: 11) introduces the notion of the "clinical" approach to inquiry.

> What do I mean by clinical? For purposes of this essay I will mean those helping professionals who get involved with individuals, groups, communities, or organisations in a "helping role". This would include clinical and counselling psychologists, psychiatrists, social workers, organisation development consultants, process consultants and others who work explicitly with human systems. I refer to trained professionals, not amateurs, so there is implied in my use of the concept of the "clinical perspective" the notion that the person has been educated and trained to take this perspective.

There are two key assumptions underlying Schein's notion of clinical inquiry. The first is that clinicians work from models of health and therefore are trained to recognise pathological deviations from health. The second assumption is that clinicians are not only concerned with diagnosis but have a primary focus on treatment.

With respect to organisations as task and social systems, what does it mean to say that such a system is "healthy"? Schein (1980) draws on the field of mental health to describe the combination of four factors of systemic health which must be present to some degree:

1. A sense of identity, purpose or mission.
2. A capacity on the part of the system to adapt and maintain itself in the face of changing internal and external circumstances.
3. A capacity to perceive and test reality.
4. Some internal integration or alignment of subsystems that make up the total system.

In a similar vein, Beckhard (1997a) highlights a strong sensing system for receiving information, a strong sense of purpose and vision of the future, structures which facilitate the work to be done, team management at the top, respect for client service as a principle, an information-driven management approach, decision making at a level closest to the client, open communication, congruent reward systems, explicit recognition for innovation and creativity, a high tolerance for different styles of thinking and ambiguity, and finally working in a learning mode where identifying learning points is part of the process of all decision making.

The clinical approach, therefore, focuses on diagnosing and treating organisational dysfunctions and pathologies. Schein (1997) outlines six clinical activities:

1. In-depth observation of crucial cases of learning and change.

2. Studying the effects of interventions.
3. Focusing on pathologies and post-mortems as a way of building a theory of health.
4. Focusing on puzzles and anomalies that are difficult to explain.
5. Building theory and empirical knowledge through developing concepts that capture the real dynamics of the organisation.
6. Focusing on the characteristics of systems and systemic dynamics.

In the context of healthcare organisations the clinical approach provides the frame on which clinicians' professional clinical knowledge and their direct experience of how the organisation actually functions can be brought together as preunderstanding on which inquiry as to how to comprehend and treat organisations can be based (Cooklin, 1999; Coghlan, 2002).

Appreciative Inquiry

The basis of appreciative inquiry takes a counter view to that of clinical inquiry. Appreciative inquiry is an approach within organisation development and action research which focuses on the best of "what is" in a system, rather than on problems to be solved, and works at engaging organisational members in envisioning and realising its future. It has been growing considerably both in academic status and practitioner application over the past few years. There is an increasing literature – books, papers, postgraduate dissertations and organisational experiences – becoming available and the major OD texts have now included it as a significant expression of contemporary OD (Cooperrider et al. 2000; Watkins and Mohr, 2001).

Appreciative inquiry is built around four phases:

1. *Discovery*: appreciating the best of "what is".
2. *Dream*: envisioning "what could be".
3. *Design*: co-constructing "what should be".
4. *Destiny*: sustaining "what will be".

Reed et al. (2002) describe an action research project in which a number of agencies and groups, including older people, engaged in an appreciative inquiry process on the subject of discharge from hospital. The positive aspect of practice as reflected through the appreciative inquiry approach contributed to inter-agency working in a blame-free environment and the involvement of service users and providers as co-researchers.

Reflective Practice

Reflective practice refers to how individuals engage in critical reflection on their own action (Schon, 1983). It involves learning to stand back from your routine practice and look at it in the light of awareness or insight.

Journal keeping is a significant tool for developing reflective skills. It involves noting your observations and experiences in a notebook and over time learning to differentiate between experiences and ways of dealing with them (Raelin, 2000). There are many useful ways of structuring a journal and your reflections. One such structure is Kolb's (1984) experiential learning cycle with the headings, experience, reflective observation, abstract conceptualisation and active experimentation. Another is Taylor's (2000) constructing, deconstructing, confronting and reconstructing.

Reflective practice is increasingly being advocated and promoted within nursing and professional practice within the health system (Ochieng, 1999; Page and Meerabeau, 2000). It is seen as a central mechanism of professional development and practice (PDP). In the context of OD, the development of reflective practice is an important and useful mechanism for individual development, which itself is valuable to organisational change.

Central to our adoption of action research, and in particular the clinical inquiry approach in this book is the process of doing action research in your own system, whether that be in your own unit, professional group or organisation. Being an inside action researcher involves learning to be able to build on the strengths of being an insider, especially knowing and having access to how things work, creating distance by standing back to inquire into what goes on and reflect on it in the light of experience and theory, and working at making improvements and change (Coghlan, 2001; Coghlan and Brannick, 2001; Coghlan and Casey, 2001; Coghlan, 2002).

ACTION RESEARCH THROUGH GROUPWORK

OD practitioners frequently utilise group approaches in their engagement in OD and action research work in organisations. These groups are the forum for shared reflection on experience and engage in the action research cycles of identifying issues, diagnosing possible causes, planning action, taking action and evaluating that action. It is becoming increasingly common to use action learning as a vehicle within OD. This next section introduces three approaches to engaging in action research and OD through a group process.

Action Learning

One common and well-established approach to organisational learning is action learning. Action learning is an approach to the development of people in organisations, which takes the task as the vehicle for learning. In action learning, people work on real issues. Action learning stands as a direct challenge to fads, packaged solutions to problems and to those forces that inhibit managers in being proactive about their own learning. While the practice of action learning is demonstrated through many different approaches, two core elements are consistently in evidence. Participants work on real organisational problems that do not appear to have clear solutions and they meet on equal terms to report to one another and to discuss their problem and progress (Pedler, 1996). Revans (1998), considered to be the father of action learning, articulated two principles on which action learning is based: "There can be no learning without action and no (sober and deliberate) action without learning" (1998: 83); "[T]hose unable to change themselves cannot change what goes on around them" (1998: 85).

Marquardt (1999) proposed six distinct interactive components of action learning:

1. *A problem*: whereby complex organisational issues, which touch on different parts of the organisation and which are not amenable to expert solutions, are selected and worked on.
2. *The group*: which comprises of, typically, six to eight members who care about the problem, know something about it and have the power to implement solutions.
3. *The questioning and reflective process*: which enacts Revans' formula for learning in action learning, $L=P+Q$. Here, L stands for learning, P for programmed learning (i.e. current knowledge in use, already known, what is in books and so on) and Q for questioning.
4. *The commitment to taking action*: whereby action learning is based on the premise that no real learning takes place unless and until action is taken. Implementation, rather than recommendations to others, is central.
5. *The commitment to learning*: whereby action learning aims at going beyond merely solving immediate problems. An increase in the knowledge and capacity to better adapt to change is more important.
6. *The facilitator*: whereby action learning groups benefit from having a facilitator, that is, one who plays a variety of roles for the group – coordinator, catalyst, observer, climate setter, communication enabler learning coach, among many others.

Action learning provides a useful methodology for the development of learning in organisations and can be a valuable OD tool. Managers can establish action learning groups (called "learning sets") comprising of members who take responsibility for a particular issue and work in a reflective mode with colleagues who support and challenge them in their efforts to make continuous innovation and learn from it. Through the action learning process, participants can enact Revans' learning formula and can subject the programmed knowledge that accompanies service delivery to questioning, action and reflection, especially in how a programmed approach is implemented in a particular organisational setting.

Learning sets have been used extensively in the health services context to provide a safe and confidential environment where health service professionals can support and challenge each other in dealing with difficult challenges and problems. Some of these sets comprise of managers from the same discipline, whereas others opt for a multi-disciplinary mix of members. Almost all follow the format of having an external facilitator establish the set, and create the framework within which it will operate. The members of the set gradually become less dependent on the facilitator to guide their learning and eventually may dispense with the facilitator and continue to meet as a self-directed set.

Flint (2001), in describing the work of nursing development units in the Irish health services, refers to action learning as one of the "more imaginative and informal strategies" used for staff development.

> The staff development potential – through enhancing the spirit of enquiry, promoting leadership and assertiveness skills and so on – of projects and other practice development activities is recognised. Shadowing, networking, learning sets and team building form part of the everyday pattern of staff development. (2001: 41)

Action research and action learning have a lot in common, as well as some fundamental differences (McGill and Beaty, 1995; Sankaran, Dick, Passfield and Swepson, 2001). Both share the same values, are based on the same learning cycle and focus on learning in action. Both emphasise collaborative relationships. Action learning takes place through the learning set process; action research, while it may be undertaken alone, involves working with others. They diverge in terms of their primary aim: action learning is fundamentally an educative process with its focus on learning, while action research places its focus on research and positions itself in contrast to traditional positivist research methods. Indeed, action research may be undertaken on action learning.

Cooperative Inquiry

A more challenging approach to organisational learning is cooperative inquiry (Heron, 1996; Reason, 1998). In cooperative inquiry, people are co-researchers in that they explore together issues that interest and concern them. The purpose is a practical one: to contribute to the flourishing of individual persons and the flourishing of human communities of inquiry. Cooperative inquiry is based on the self-determining nature of the human person, which means that the co-researchers determine to a significant degree what they do and what they experience as part of the research. The participants examine their own experience in collaboration with others who share similar interests and concerns. What is significant is their critical awareness, their quality of reflection and their informed judgements, which contrasts with the unexamined projections and consensus collusion of non-critical groups.

Meehan (2001) describes how he used cooperative inquiry as a means of carrying out an evaluation of an alcohol addiction counselling service. The deliverers of the service formed a cooperative inquiry group and engaged in cycles of reflection on their experience of delivering the service and of working within their organisation and in developing new and creative ways of looking at things. They also learned to take action, to change things they wanted to change and explored how to do things better. Each member acted as a co-subject in the reflection phases and a co-researcher in the action phases. They enacted the action research cycles of action and reflection in a psychologically safe environment, which enabled them to make sense of their experience and to take steps to initiate change.

Peter Reason of Bath University provides several accounts and reflections on cooperative inquiry work in which he has engaged with health practitioners. He notes how cooperative inquiry contributes to professional practice (1998), how it is a valuable and significant approach for engaging in multi-disciplinary collaboration (1992) and provides a social setting for managing issues of power and conflict that arise in multi-disciplinary work (1991).

Parallel Learning Structures

Groups which meet to reflect on experience and work at enabling organisational learning to take place may be seen as parallel learning structures (Bushe and Shani, 1991). Parallel learning structures are those structures, such as action learning and cooperative inquiry groups, that are attending to learning processes in the organisation and that co-exist in parallel with the regular structures of the organisation. Such groups are typically engaging in subversive activity. Not that the existence or membership of the groups are secret or that what they are doing is actually subversive. What is subversive about them is that they are counter-cultural to the dominant culture of most organisations, which typically rewards focusing on individuals attending only to their own job, working within their own discipline, not raising awkward questions, particularly about process, and keeping line relations based on authority and control. What is subversive about them is that the members learn a different way of working and relating through their participation in them. The different way of working involves building peer relations across disciplines in order to inquire into organisational processes in a collaborative manner. Rather than working from the organisation's espoused theory, the focus is reflection on experience and inquiry into the organisation's theory-in-use. What becomes subversive is that out of their experiences in the groups the participants begin to influence the ways the organisation works. In effect, they subvert traditional mindsets and norms, which hitherto prevented the organisation from exposing its own ways of working to reflection and critique, and so open it up to engaging in processes of organisational double-loop learning.

An example of a parallel learning structure is a group established to develop care pathways for particular client groups referred to a service. Working together in a group comprised of several disciplines allows them the opportunity to step outside of their own profession's perspective and view the problems and blockages in the patient pathway from the perspective of the patient and of the other professions. Together this group can develop an understanding of the best way of organising the services of the different professionals in order to ensure a smooth transition through the system for the patient.

Shani and Eberhardt (1987) describe the use of a parallel structure in a US hospital where it was considered that traditional research and management methods had failed to improve healthcare team effectiveness. The parallel structure was a microcosm of the medical organisation and comprised of representatives from each of the medical professional departments, employees who were at least moderately verbal and who would be perceived as representative by their constituents, and employees who agreed voluntarily to serve on the study group. The group designed survey questionnaires, observed teams at work and interviewed personnel. It was found that many worked at a multidisciplinary level rather than an interdisciplinary level. Data from the study was fed back to the hospital employees by both management and the parallel structure group along with a list of recommended actions. The parallel structure group designed a longitudinal experimental study to assess scientifically and to compare the effectiveness of the two kinds of teams, and was charged with the responsibility of carrying out and monitoring the experiment. The hospital acquired and developed some basic learning mechanisms needed to learn about itself by itself and had a structure and process in place that could generate knowledge and recommendations for action.

CONCLUSIONS

In this chapter we have developed the notion of OD and action research as intimately intertwined. Both come from the same origin and work on the basis of an emergent and contingent approach to change, which follows repetitive cycles of diagnosis, planning, action and evaluation. We have briefly introduced a number of approaches to action research, some of which may be undertaken by individuals and some of which are group based, and we have provided illustrations of how experience can be studied with a view to both taking action and improving understanding.

Case 3.1 Dealing with Non-Attendances

Carricksimon health centre has had increasing DNA (did not attend) rates over the past twelve months. A substantial number of those failing to attend are appointments for children aged twelve and under. The issue has been discussed at several team meetings to date, but no decision has been made on what to do about the problem. The social worker on the team pointed out that there has been a significant staff turnover in the past twelve months with two psychologists being replaced and three new family therapists starting, in a team of fifteen professional staff. She feels that this must be contributing to the problem. The three general practitioners disagree, saying she is reading too much into this and it is simply that the parents have so much on their minds that they forget their children's appointments. The public health nurse feels that the location of the health centre is an issue as it is not on any main public transport route. Several months ago the administrator offered to review the files to look for patterns in the non-attendance, but she has not had the time to do so.

The issue is now being raised again because the health centre's manager has received a memo from the Health Board to say that they will shortly be conducting an efficiency review on the centre's work. All staff in the centre agree that the DNAs are creating inefficiency in the clinic and are committed to tackling the issue themselves in advance of the review.

Question
Which of the approaches outlined in the chapter would you consider most suitable to addressing this issue, and why?

Clinical Inquiry Exercise 3.1

Take a change initiative that you are currently working on that has become stuck or is progressing slower than expected.

1. Using a clinical inquiry approach try to identify, through post-mortems of recent meetings and events, the puzzles and anomalies that are difficult to explain.

cont/d

2. When you are comfortable with this approach, try it out with the group involved in implementing the change.
3. Can you find a way of "unsticking" progress through such clinical inquiry?

PART II

UNDERSTANDING
ORGANISATIONS

Chapter 4

Organisations as Systems

The notion of organisations is an abstraction. It is a concept that helps us grasp the complexity of collective organisation and action. So when we say that we work for the hospital we do not mean the building in a specific location that has signs identifying it, but rather that we work for the collective entity that is a legal term and has legal, structural and psychological associations attached to it. This chapter addresses ways of looking at organisations.

There are many ways of understanding organisations. We may be familiar with different approaches within organisation theory that emphasise institution (institutional theory), resources (resource-dependency theory) or the environment (population ecology). A common approach is to think of organisations in terms of metaphors – machine, organism, culture, political system, brain and psychic prison (Morgan, 1997). However one approaches the notion of an organisation, one is attempting to grasp a complex abstraction. In this chapter we describe and explore the systems approach, first in general and second through the particular systems lens which is the Burke-Litwin model.

UNDERSTANDING ORGANISATIONS AS SYSTEMS

Systems thinking refers to seeing organisations as a whole, made up of interrelated and interdependent parts, with the whole being more than the sum of its parts. The human body is a good example of a system, whereby bones, muscles, tissues and organs are not simply a collection of these items as in a shopping bag but perform interdependent and interrelated functions. While we might dissect the body and make an analysis of any particular part, an understanding of the body's functioning depends on a holistic view of how all the parts work together. Similarly, organisations may be viewed as systems, in which planning, control, structural, technological and behavioural systems are interdependent and interrelated.

Organisations are understood to be open systems, by which is meant that they are dependent on and in continual interaction with their external environment for their survival (Burke, 2002). Living systems are "open systems" as they depend on taking in oxygen and food from the environment; mechanical systems are "closed systems" because they function within themselves. Health organisations are open systems as they are responsive to the health of the nation and dependent on the work and skills of people who are recruited into them. The expertise of employees and the available technology together are transformed to deliver a healthcare service, the output of which contributes to or feeds back into the health of the nation.

A second way we might understand organisations as systems is through the "recursive" systems model, which represents organisations as patterns of feedback loops and sequences of interaction that link and integrate elements of a system (Senge, 1990; Senge et al. 1994, 1999; McCaughan and Palmer, 1994; Pratt, Gordon and Plamping, 1999). Feedback refers to any reciprocal flow of influence (Senge, 1990). So we might think of traffic as a recursive system. We know from experience of traffic problems that it is not enough to say that the congestion is caused by too many cars on the road (A is causing B) but that the number of cars on the road is also influenced by the state of public transport, the size of roads, public policy, parking facilities, people's attitudes to city travel, the current state of the economy, all of which interact over time in a series of complex loops, each being a cause and effect of the other. Each of these elements provides feedback and sets off a reaction. So if people find public transport unreliable they take their car into the city, which over time increases congestion and contributes to the unreliability of public transport. Traffic planners and public policy makers must take the systemic nature of traffic into consideration and attempt to make interventions that address the complexity of the system. In systems thinking, linear cause and effect analysis is replaced by viewing patterns of interaction that mutually influence each other.

If we look at the health system we can also see these patterns of interaction. A contentious issue for many health systems is waiting times for elective treatment. The "congestion" in the health system, just as the traffic congestion, cannot be accounted for solely by the increasing numbers of patients requiring treatment. The number of beds available and how these beds are currently utilised will influence the throughput, which in turn will influence waiting times. The range and complexity of diseases and procedures will also play a role, with more complex procedures generally requiring more time and resources. Seasonal influences play a part, with cold weather leading to increasing ill health in the elderly, which in turn increases demand for beds. In some areas the tourist season means a substantial increase in the population and increased attendance at accident and emergency departments. This can place strain on regular services and result in the cancellation of elective cases in some instances. If this happens over a prolonged period, it may lead to a backlog that further lengthens the waiting lists. The retention of staff, which may be influenced by how "healthy" the organisation is externally perceived to be, can also influence throughput and in turn waiting times. The general health of the population, the investment of resources in preventive strategies and primary care and the emergence of epidemics of disease are also factors that can influence demand over time. In such a complex system of interacting forces it is clear that addressing one issue may not be enough to solve the problem.

Many writers on systems thinking refer to the "shift of mind" that is necessary to engage in systems thinking (Senge, 1990; Owen and Lambert, 1995). One way of thinking about the world is that there is an external reality "out there" and that "we" are independent of that reality. However, in systems thinking "we" and "our behaviour" must be recognised as an integral part of the whole, such that our behaviour affects reality and reality affects our behaviour.

"Dynamic complexity" refers to situations where a system is complex, not because of a lot of detail but because of multiple causes and effects over time (Senge, 1990). In situations of dynamic complexity, systems thinking provides a perspective of viewing and understanding how a system is held together by patterns of action and reaction, relationships, meanings and hidden rules, and the role of time. This approach is central to the work of family therapists and the constructs from family therapy have been adapted to organisational consultation (Bor and Miller, 1991; Campbell, Draper and Huffington, 1991; Campbell, Coldicott and Kinsella, 1994).

Mintzberg (1997) writes about hospitals as "disconnected" systems or systems in which the sub-systems remain largely disconnected from each other. Mintzberg refers to the "four worlds" in a hospital. He argues that some people manage down – straight into the operations in question, to the direct delivery of service; some manage up – dealing largely with the authorities above them and people outside of the system; while others manage out – to people not quite so formally committed to it. Mintzberg labels these worlds as care (inhabited by nurses), cure (inhabited by doctors), control (inhabited by managers) and community (inhabited by hospital board members). Because of the different perspectives of these four groups and the disconnectedness between their worlds, fragmentation occurs, making it difficult to manage the delivery of a seamless service.

Campbell, Coldicott and Kinsella (1994) argue that the problems faced by many change and effectiveness improvement programmes is the positivist-oriented approach that pushes people towards trying to "discover" the "best way" to improve an organisation. This approach, they argue, is underpinned by the assumption that "local" difficulties can be solved through the application of "universal" good practice. Hence there is a tendency to look outwards for solutions. Systems thinking is useful in that it ensures that the organisation looks inwards as well as outwards and systems approaches tend to remove blame from the picture and instead focus on cause and effect. Campbell et al. (1994) suggest that introducing systemic thinking to an organisation requires a paradigm shift:

Away from		Towards
"solve the problem"	➤	"create the future"
"bring in the expert"	➤	"help people learn"
"identify the accountable manager"	➤	"involve everybody"
"find the right technique"	➤	"find a helpful process"
"find the best way"	➤	"find a better way"
"get a quick fix"	➤	"improve continuously"

In keeping with this paradigm shift, Campbell et al. identify a set of useful criteria for systemic consultation in large organisations. We draw on these shifts or criteria to develop a systemic consulting approach with health organisations.

1. *Universal to local.* The gap between management intent and local practice needs to be bridged. It is essential that opportunities are created for meaningful interaction between these levels. In the case of a health strategy that has been developed at the top levels, the implementation of this strategy is dependent on the translation of the vision and goals into practical steps that can be followed at the service-delivery level.

2. *Observed to observing systems.* We are all part of the system we operate in and therefore part of any problems or diagnoses – nobody, not even the CEO, is an independent observer or a victim of something happening "out there" or in "senior management". The "observed" system phenomenon classically manifests itself in the "them" and "us" scenarios that exist in the health system – between management and doctors, between senior management and more junior managers, between front line managers and their staff, and between health board management and the Department of Health and Children. The flexibility of the organisation and its ability to adapt can be enhanced significantly if members of the organisation at every level can connect their own actions with others' reactions.

3. *Part to whole.* Working with wide representation from the system in planning the change will lead to greater commitment and less resistance in the implementation of the change, a point we made in chapter 2 with the National Health Strategy.

4. *Debate to dialogue.* Inquiry through dialogue is likely to generate

more alternative options for change or problem solving than the traditional debating approach. Moving away from a compartmentalised approach to a more inclusive one that utilises expertise from the wider organisation leads to more creativity in problem solving. The resolution of a problem that occurs in the A&E department may benefit from involvement of staff from other departments as there is interconnectedness between what happens in A&E and other parts of the hospital.

5. *Detail to dynamic complexity.* Change leadership is more effective when focusing on the meanings in a dynamic system rather than focusing on detailing the processes. Individual and shared perceptions create the organisation's reality and explain "how we do things around here". Documenting detailed processes is not sufficient to change behaviours, as is evidenced by the failure of BPR approaches to change the culture of hospitals (Bate, 2000a).

6. *Quantification to appreciation.* This follows from the previous point in saying that attention to quantitative measurement will not help to control a complex organisation. This is particularly true for healthcare organisations where the reactions of skilled professionals to simplistic performance measures is difficult to predict. It is far better to try to appreciate what performance means to organisational members.

7. *Instructive to interactive.* Interactive learning or action learning is much more likely to lead to changes in practice than purely instructive learning. We are all too familiar with this scenario in healthcare where resources are continually invested in short training courses for managers at similar levels or grades, with such training frequently being divorced from the context of managers' daily work lives. Such training activity may lead to a burst of enthusiasm from the individual manager, but this is invariably short lived when the manager returns to the work context and finds that colleagues do not share this "new" view of the world that he/she has discovered.

8. *Instruments to processes of management.* There is an endless search for instruments that will identify better managers and tools that will help us to manage better. The health system has recently adopted the concept of "core competencies" or essential skills to guide the recruitment and training of healthcare managers. Campbell et al. (1994) argue that competencies describe "behaviour in relationships", not individual behaviour in isolation, and as such their meaning is socially created through the process of people agreeing on their experience of an event.

9. *Literal to oral communication.* Ong (1982) bemoans the "technologizing" of the word communication and claims it has lead to the demise of our oral heritage. Campbell et al. (1994) write about "pipeline" communication of "packages" of facts. The transmission of the message needs to take account of the context and anticipate the feedback. The oral means is the best in achieving this.

10. *Espousal to enactment.* Enacting change does not occur through espousal of vision and ideas alone. Change or enactment of that vision needs to be evident in leaders' behaviour. Complex change requires the adoption of new behaviours by staff at all levels and in their interactions and relationships with each other. Practice what we preach must be the motto.

Thinking in terms of systems means (Anderson and Johnson, 1997):

- *Thinking of the big picture.* This means standing back from the immediate focus and looking at the patterns of the bigger picture. This can sometimes mean looking beyond the health system at other environmental influences on health. For example, if we are to stem the increasing demand for health services we need to look at ways of influencing poverty and health education.

- *Balancing long- and short-term perspectives.* Systems show that short-term success often hurts in the long term. For example developing a rostering arrangement to try to please all the staff on the ward and accommodate everyone's holidays this year may result in a very happy and productive group of staff in the short term. However, if the ward manager has not paid attention to the knock-on implications of next year's holidays, he/she may find that he/she is paying for his/her generosity by creating an expectation that staff will always be accommodated to take their holidays when they choose.

- *Recognizing the dynamic, complex and interdependent nature of systems.* As explored in the traffic and waiting-list examples above, simplification and linear thinking have their limitations.

- *Taking into account both measurable and non-measurable factors.* Some data are measurable, such as the length of hospital stay or overall bed occupancy of a hospital. Other factors are not measurable, such as the exact contribution of each aspect of a patient's treatment to the recovery of that patient. For example, in a patient who suffered from depression we cannot be certain whether the anti-depressants or the psychotherapy had the greatest effect for that individual. We can only look at evidence from research of similar groups of people suffering from depression, or we can measure the patient's own perception of what was most helpful or indeed seek the opinion of the different health professionals involved. However, none of these give us a clear measure. This does not mean that the data is irrelevant. Systems thinking encourages the use of both kinds of data.

- *Remember that we are all part of the systems in which we function and that we influence those systems even as we are being influenced by them.* Our ways of thinking about issues (what Senge (1990) calls "mental models") influence our actions which influence others. For example, if a hospital manager views the concept of involving clinicians in management as a directive from the Department of Health and Children and not necessarily something that will make a difference to patient care, she is likely to postpone discussions on this every time something more pertinent arises. Continuous postponement gives the strong message that this issue is not high priority for hospital management. This in turn may dampen any enthusiasm that exists amongst the clinical staff, as they may believe there is little chance of implementing a new structure. There are often unintended consequences to managerial actions. For example, a head physiotherapist may reward one of her staff for her contribution to the development of the department by funding her to go to a conference. She may then unexpectedly find herself faced with a request from the union to explain why there is inequity in conference funding for staff.

In order to inquire into how a system functions, OD practitioners can engage in systemic questioning (McCaughan and Palmer, 1994):

- *Establishing circuitry*: Does one event trigger another?
- *Establishing patterns*: What patterns are evident over time? What does A do? What does B do in response? What does A do next? Is there seasonal variation? What are the typical patterns that repeat annually?
- *Exploring meaning*: What are the meanings held in the system? What are the common meanings attributed to their actions?
- *Exploring covert rules*: What unarticulated and hidden rules govern behaviour? Do not discuss passive regressive retaliation.
- *Exploring the time dimensions*: How time delays have an impact on the system.
- *Formulation of tentative working explanations as to what is happening in the system*: The circuitry, patterns, covert rules, meanings and time may uncover the dynamic complexity of the system, and may involve many iterations of collaborative inquiry before finding explanations that fit.

Case 4.1 Chaotic Outpatient Clinic

A multi-disciplinary team exploring the reason for a chaotic outpatient clinic at first decided the clerks were at fault because they operate a system that means only one clerk is acting as receptionist at any point in time. On delving deeper the team found that there was overbooking of patients in the clinics (*establishing circuitry*). Further iterations of the inquiry revealed that certain consultants allow their clinics to over-run on a regular basis. On examining which consultants and on what days, patterns emerged to suggest that when consultant A runs into consultant B's clinic, then consultant B over-books patients for clinics he holds immediately before consultant A in a deliberate attempt to over-run into A's clinics (*establishing patterns*). Further examination showed that these over-runs happen at the same time every month. Discussions with the clerks revealed that these are the days that pharmaceutical representatives visit the clinic and that they upset the clinic by spending unscheduled time with the consultants (*exploring meaning*). Examination of the rosters revealed that there are more agency nursing staff scheduled on these same days. Discussions with nursing management revealed that there are high sickness and absenteeism rates on these days (*exploring covert rules*). Could it be that some nurses knowing that clinics will over-run by up to two hours on these days, become ill when they find that they are scheduled to be on duty in these clinics? (*exploring meaning and time dimensions*)

Case 4.1 serves to highlight the value of repeated iterations of collaborative inquiry. With each iteration we collect more data until we begin to build the complex picture of the factors that are contributing to the particular problem.

A very useful way of formulating systemic explanations is through the use of diagrammatic representation. When cycles of action and their consequences are drawn in a diagram, the patterns of the system may be illuminated. Both the act of attempting to represent the system diagrammatically and the diagram itself are essential elements of the learning process. The very act of drawing the system's diagram is a learning process of explanation formulation and testing (Anderson and Johnson, 1997). The systems approach holds the key to integrating intuition and reason, because intuition goes beyond linear thinking to recognise patterns, draw analogies and solve problems. Figure 4.1 is a diagrammatic representation of the Chaotic Outpatient clinic inquiry. Representing it diagrammatically helps to map out potential points for intervention.

Figure 4.1 Chaotic Outpatient Clinic

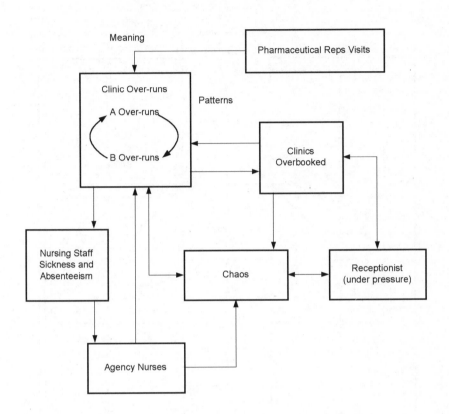

THE BURKE-LITWIN CAUSAL MODEL OF ORGANISATION PERFORMANCE AND CHANGE

The Burke-Litwin model provides an organisation framework that helps explain open systems theory in action and provides a way of thinking about planned organisation change (Burke and Litwin, 1992; Burke, 2002) (Figure 4.2). Looking at the very top and bottom of the model (overleaf), the external environment box serves as the input dimension to the organisation, while the individual and organisational performance box serves as the output dimension. The boxes in between provide the transformation dimensions. The arrows illustrate the recursive feedback loops. As Burke points out, to portray the model as close to reality as possible there would be arrows connecting all the boxes, but the figure does not do that in order to avoid making the diagram too daunting and messy. The model predicts cause, so some directions are more important than others in planning and implementing organisation change.

Figure 4.2 The Burke-Litwin Model of Organisational Performance and Change

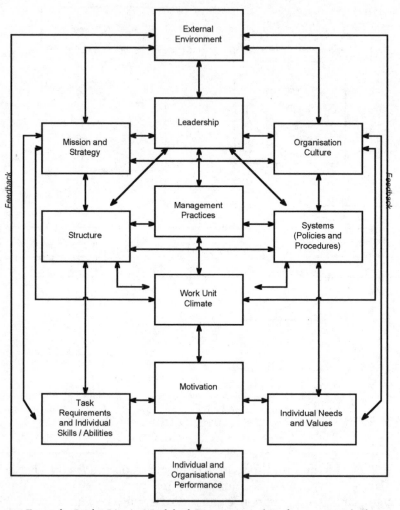

Source: From the Burke-Litwin Model of Organisational Performance and Change.
© 1987, 1992 by W. Warner Burke, Associates Inc. Reproduced with permission.

The key to understanding the model is to compare the top half with the bottom half. The boxes in the top half – external environment, mission and strategy, leadership and culture – are termed *transformational* factors, i.e. those that bring about change in the entire organisation. The boxes in the lower half – management practices, structure, systems, work-unit climate, motivation, individual needs and values, task requirements – are termed *transactional* factors and are concerned with day-to-day operations, continuous improvement and evolutionary change. Change in transformational factors requires change leadership while change in transactional factors requires managers who focus on improvement.

We now discuss each factor in turn and apply the Burke-Litwin model to healthcare systems.

Transformational Factors

The transformational factors are those that immediately respond to the external environment forces. Mission and strategy set the fundamental identity and direction of the organisation, are shaped and led by leaders and are enabled or inhibited by organisational culture (Figure 4.3).

Figure 4.3 The Transformational Factors

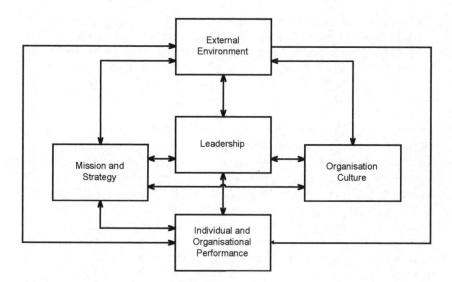

External Environment
The external environment refers to those forces or changes taking place outside of the organisation that will influence organisational performance. The political climate for example has a direct impact on health systems, particularly in the time period immediately before an election when health moves up the political agenda. Political priorities, not health priorities may result in the postponement of a planned hospital closure, or may work to the organisation's advantage if it finds itself moved up the list of priority projects for capital investment. Changing legislation is another external factor that can impact on health. For example the 1997 Freedom of Information Act which allows a) members of the public the right to

obtain access to official information and b) the information commissioner conduct reviews of decisions of public bodies in relation to requests for access to information, had a major impact on record keeping and on the transparency of decision making in healthcare organisations. The economic climate also has significant implications as it determines the size of the health budget, which in turn influences levels of activity, numbers of posts that can be filled and so on. Public scandals have the potential to impact negatively on health organisations, a prime example being the hepatitis C caused by blood transfusions, which lead to a dramatic fall in blood donations.

Mission and Strategy

Mission is the term used to describe the organisation's *raison d'être*, and answers the question "Why does this organisation exist?" It refers to the present and clearly sets out the purpose of the organisation in a brief statement. The Department of Health and Children's mission statement is:

> In a partnership with the providers of health care, and in co-operation with other government departments, statutory and non-statutory bodies, to protect, promote and restore the well-being of the people by ensuring the health and personal social services are planned, managed and delivered to achieve measurable health and social gain and provide the optimum return on resources invested. (http://www.doh.ie)

This mission statement has a clear focus on the desired outputs and outcomes, whilst also acknowledging the various inputs that are required to achieve these outcomes. The use of the words "protect, promote and restore" gives the clear message that the Department considers its remit to be broader than the treatment of disease and is focused on the provision of a health service not just a healthcare service, i.e. not just restoring health but preventing ill health arising in the first place. Significant words such as "cooperation" and "measurable" have been carefully chosen to indicate the change of emphasis in how the Department plans to do business.

Strategy follows from mission in that it sets out how the organisation or system will accomplish its mission over the next three to five years. Many strategic development initiatives begin not just with a mission but also a vision. Vision differs from mission in that it refers to the future and gives a picture of where the organisation would like to be. It usually contains phrases that suggest a challenge for the organisation. Common examples in healthcare include "to be a centre of excellence for the treatment of cancer", "to provide the best care", "to obtain satisfaction ratings greater than 95%", "to be the best teaching hospital in the city" and so on. The Health Strategy (2001: 8) sets out a very simple but powerful vision of:

A health system that:

- supports and empowers you, your family and community to achieve your full health potential
- is there when you need it, that is fair and that you can trust
- encourages you to have your say, listens to you, ensures that your views are taken into account.

This is clearly a challenge to a system that currently has major access difficulties, where trust has been eroded by repeated public scandals and for which there is a question about the fairness of a system that has a public–private mix.

The Health Strategy, *Quality and Fairness: A Health System for You*, sets out how this vision will be achieved following through from the vision to identify four national goals:

1. Better health for everyone.
2. Fair access.
3. Responsive and appropriate care delivery.
4. High performance.

The frameworks to deliver these goals included strengthening primary care and reforming the acute hospital system. So we can see in the strategy a logical progression from where we are now towards the vision that has been painted.

It has only really been in the past six to seven years that healthcare organisations in Ireland have devoted attention to strategy development. Prior to this they were almost exclusively focused on operational issues and the planning was seen as the domain of the Department of Health and Children. The absence of strategy in healthcare organisations prior to this may in part account for the persistence of the mechanistic, bureaucratic organisation in situations where it was no longer in fit with the purpose or mission of the organisation. Change was for the most part focused on management practices, structures and systems whilst the transformational factors such as mission and strategy, and leadership and organisational culture were left untouched.

Leadership

An important distinction is made between leaders and managers (Zaleznik, 1977; Carney, 1999; Fedoruk and Pincombe, 2000). Leaders provide vision, direction and energy towards change; they influence people by acting as a role model, by encouragement and praise, and they generate enthusiasm and excitement. Managers function more within a role. They work within the organisation's objectives and use resources and information efficiently and effectively. While the two overlap, they are treated separately in this model. Leadership as a transformational factor refers to the behaviour of senior executives and managers throughout the organisation who provide direction and positive energy for change. We will focus on leadership and leading change in chapter 9.

Exploring the difference between management and leadership at ward level, one would expect a managerially focused ward manager to be concerned about bed occupancy, throughput, staffing levels, expenditure and average lengths of stay. A ward manager with more leadership ability would probably be more concerned with benchmarking performance against other wards, with improving organisational culture and climate, and developing innovations that might also be utilised in other wards. A simplistic but relevant difference is that leaders will tend to be more outwardly focused, whereas managers tend to be more inwardly focused.

Culture

When people talk about what organisational culture is, they typically see it as "the way we do things around here". When we read the popular literature about organisational culture we find it speaks of climate, becoming a learning organisation or building a team-based culture, and hence it often focuses on human relations issues, such as communication and teamwork. These are essential elements of culture but are not the total picture. Organisational culture is a complex reality. We do not see culture because it is too close to us. It only comes into consciousness when it is challenged, as when we go to another organisation or we have new members in our own organisation.

Schein (1999a) describes three levels of culture which go from the visible to the invisible or. The first level is the *artefact* level. These are the visible things – what we see, hear and feel as we visit an organisation – the visible layout of the office, whether people work with their door open or closed, how people are dressed, how people treat one another, how meetings are conducted, how disagreements or conflicts are handled and so on. The difficulty about these visible artefacts is that they are hard to decipher. We do not know why people behave this way or why things are this way. When we ask these questions we get the official answers, the answers that present the values that the organisation wants to portray. This is the second level of culture – *organisational values*. Open doors are a sign of open communication and teamwork; first name greetings are a sign of informality – this sort of thing. Yet we know that this is not always true; that organisations, not unlike individuals, do not always live up to what they espouse, not necessarily due to any deliberate, nefarious or conspiratorial reason to deceive but for complex, unknown, hidden reasons. A more common answer to our question is more likely to be, "I do not know; they did things this way long before I joined and I got the message early on that this is how we do things here." So we come to the third level of culture: *shared tacit assumptions*. These are the assumptions which have grown up in the organisation and which have made it successful. They are typically tacit or hidden because they have been passed from generation to generation within an organisation and organisation members do not see them any more because they are taken for granted.

Therefore, culture is much deeper than open doors, plants and bright colours, and mission statements and strategic plans. When we look at initiatives and why they have not worked or achieved their intended outcomes, the answer is likely to be that the initiatives violate some taken-for-granted assumptions that are embedded in the organisational psyche because they were successful in the past. That is the key. Because something is successful at some point in time it gets passed on as "the way we do things around here". Schein (1999a: 29) sees culture as "the sum total of all the taken-for-granted assumptions that a group has learned through its history." Therefore, an organisation's culture is deep – it controls us more than we control it. It is broad and it is stable as it sets predictability and normality, and hence changing it evokes anxiety and resistance.

While the notion of culture is abstract, it is also very concrete. There is no right or wrong, better or worse culture. These are judgements that can only be made in terms of what an organisation is trying to do. Appropriate or inappropriate culture only makes sense in the context of what a particular organisation is trying to do and what assumptions an organisation needs to hold to be successful in its environment.

How do we assess our organisation's culture? This is difficult because we do not know what to ask about our own culture. So questionnaires do not tell us much about the organisation's culture. As culture is concretely embedded it can be uncovered through reflecting on how concrete issues are handled. So a group could take a concrete problem or something it would like to improve or make work better. The group might find it useful to review the concept of culture existing at the three different levels of artefacts, espoused values and shared tacit assumptions. Then the group could work at identifying lots of artefacts that characterise the organisation. Then it could name the organisation's espoused values as published in missions and policy statements. Finally the group might compare the espoused values with the artefacts in those same areas.

Applying Schein's levels of culture to performance management:

- What are the artefacts of performance management? They are the stated policies, the inclusion of performance indicators in service plans, the use of competency-based interviewing and so on.
- The values espoused are those enshrined in strategy and the new legislation and regulations governing the public service, accountability, transparency, the norms for customer service and so on.

- What are the shared tacit assumptions that prevent it from being implemented effectively? We do not blame individuals for being traditionalist, old fashioned or stuck-in-the-mud. We know that people who find performance management difficult do so because they have been socialised into another way of working. Singling out individuals for reward or criticism will have a negative influence on staff morale. In the past there were other ways of doing things that were based on shared tacit assumptions, which were successful both for the organisation and for the individuals in it. What were those assumptions? People helped each other. The performance of the team was more important than the performance of the individual. How is it that they do not apply anymore?

What are the important elements of forming culture in a new organisation? Schein declares that the primary mechanisms that embed culture in a new organisation are found in the behaviour of the leaders. What do they pay attention to, measure and control regularly? How do they react to critical incidents and organisational crises? What criteria do they use to allocate scarce resources? What behaviours do they role model? If organisational leaders are the primary sources of culture, then efforts to develop leadership skills are an essential strategy in cultural change.

But leadership behaviour is not enough by itself; it needs to be supported by other organisational mechanisms. Some secondary mechanisms that embed culture are the structure of the organisation, the systems and procedures, the rituals, the design of psychical space, the stories and legends that are told about people and events, and probably least the statements of organisational philosophy and mission. Take teamwork for example. An organisation may espouse teamwork, i.e. it says it wants people to work together, to share information and be co-responsible and co-accountable. At the same time, performance is measured individually and ultimately promotion is based on individual work and, perhaps, individual work that is achieved at the expense of others. Hence the message goes around, "What really matters here is individual work", and so the espoused focus on teamwork is actually negated by existing, more powerful structures. To take another example, the organisational values espouse clarity, but the tacit shared assumptions may be that seeking clarity gets you into trouble and that keeping things close to your chest or deliberately vague is rewarded. Consequently, efforts to develop clarity get nowhere.

In short we do not examine culture in the abstract. We try to see what shared tacit assumptions are operative in a concrete issue. Schein thinks that to do this kind of work a group probably needs an external facilitator who can ask questions and help the group stand back from what it does not know it knows. This is not to say that we might need a facilitator who is external to the organisation, but rather that we might use one who is external to the unit or the team but internal to the service. Hence there is great importance in having OD skills in house.

Transactional Factors

The transactional factors represent those organisational domains that concern day-to-day operations, incremental and evolutionary change (Figure 4.4).

Figure 4.4 The Transactional Factors

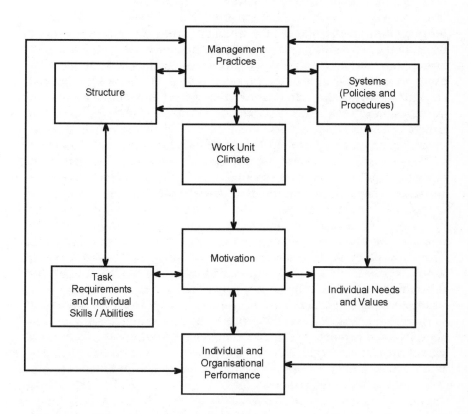

Structure
Organisational structure refers to the way an organisation is structured in terms of functions (departments) and reporting relationships, and is usually represented by an organisational chart consisting of boxes with job titles and solid or broken connecting lines. It is a useful representation of levels of authority, lines of responsibility and pathways of communication within an organisation. Changing an organisation's

structure is a transactional rather than a transformational factor for change, because a structural change that involves moving people into different roles and changing titles will not necessarily create revolutionary change in an organisation. It could be likened to "moving deck-chairs on the Titanic", i.e. it would not prevent the ship from sinking.

There has been a considerable amount of structural change in the health system in recent years. Closer examination of these changes shows that structural change is more successful in achieving the aims of the organisation when it is accompanied by other changes. For example, the change in hospital structures that introduced clinical directorates has met with varying degrees of success but seems to be more successful where new personnel in the form of business managers/or nurse managers have been recruited, as they have been instrumental in introducing new ways of organising the work of the specialty. Also the change from a programme structure to a "care group" structure in many of the health boards has been difficult for some because of the lack of planning expertise within the new care-group structures. The significant structural change in the health services for the eastern region has seen the introduction of the Eastern Regional Health Authority. This major structural change has been accompanied by a change in emphasis from "planning based on dictate" to "planning based on comprehensive needs assessment" and from overseeing through "budget control" to overseeing through "regular monitoring and evaluation". Without these changes the structural change alone would not have resulted in more integrated services in the eastern region.

Management Practices
This box addresses how managers behave on a day-to-day basis to achieve organisation goals. We know that managers can behave in many different ways, from autocratic bullying at one extreme to opt out, non-involvement at the other. Managers frequently present their leadership dilemmas in terms of a tension between the task of the group and their concern for the individuals in the group. They find, in some cases, that what benefits the group task may not be to the benefit of the individuals in the group, and vice versa. This is undoubtedly true in some instances. As managers have a responsibility for getting the job done and for looking after the welfare of their personnel as part of the description of their role, a framework that takes account of both is useful in the Leadership Grid® which is described in chapter 9.

Systems
Systems refer to the procedures that are in place that help to accomplish the tasks of the organisation. Patient information systems, service planning as a system of resource allocation and human resource management systems such as personal development planning are all

examples of systems that facilitate the work of healthcare organisations. Although the introduction of a new system such as performance appraisal may gradually lead to change in an organisation, partly as a result of the knock-on effects on culture and possibly leadership, a new system introduced in isolation will not lead to immediate transformational change. An effective performance appraisal system should improve individual performance and may improve team performance, depending on how contribution to teamwork is appraised. This in turn may gradually lead to improved inter-team working and the organisation may slowly begin to shift from a "blame and shame" culture to a "recognition and reward culture".

Climate

Climate is the collective perceptions of people within the same team, department or work group. Perceptions regarding how they are managed, how clear they are about their manager's expectations of them, how valued they believe their contributions are, how much support they receive, how involved in decision making they feel and how well they believe they work with other parts of the organisation.

Let us explore the climate of a psychology department that invited an OD consultant to help build team morale, when it was raised at a department meeting that morale had fallen considerably in the past year. The OD facilitator, through discussions with individual staff and sub-groups of the department, surfaced a whole plethora of phrases that are relevant to diagnosing the climate of the department. A few examples:

- "Our head of department is never here, he's always off to one committee or another."
- "Those psychiatrists are undermining our work by changing medication regimes during our clients' therapy."
- "Community psychiatric nurses seem to be a law unto themselves taking direct referrals from general practitioners and running therapy groups, and the community services general manager just stands back and says nothing."
- "We are inundated with referrals…nobody listens when we point out that the department needs more staff…and my colleagues spend so much time moaning about how awful the pressure is, that I find it impossible to achieve the goals I set myself."
- "I suppose you've [OD consultant] been sent to empower us…well we cannot change the situation because nobody tells us what is happening in this organisation."

Clearly this climate is not conducive to a highly motivated team delivering an effective service. This climate may be indicative of an organisational culture in which inter-group collaboration is not seen as important in the achievement of the organisation's goals and some professions are given a higher value than others. It may equally be a localised climate that has been created in large part by the head of department's leadership style. Improving the climate of this department will almost certainly improve the morale and productivity of its members. However, whether it results in significant change in the organisation as a whole is very much dependent on the factors at a higher level that may or may not be influencing the existing climate.

Task Requirements and Job Skills

This refers to the degree to which there is congruence between the requirements of an individual's job and that individual's competencies to fulfil those requirements. For example, an organisation providing services for people with disabilities has difficulty recruiting speech and language therapists and finds itself having to offer a head of department post to a therapist who has three years post-qualification experience in a general community speech and language therapist's post. Whilst this person is an excellent therapist she has no experience of disability services, nor has she any managerial training or expertise. She may well experience considerable stress in her new role because of these personal shortcomings. This could result not only in her individual performance being poor, but also the performance of the service as a whole.

The health service has recently shifted the focus of recruitment and interviewing practices from valuing knowledge of the health system and years and breadth of experience to valuing the competencies that are pertinent to the job to which the person is being recruited. Also staff development tends to be more competency based than was previously the case.

Individual Needs and Values

Most behavioural scientists believe that enriched jobs enhance motivation. If individuals' needs and values are congruent with the organisation's values this is likely to lead to a more motivated workforce and improved performance. In health systems it is argued that health professionals' values are for the most part congruent with the health system's goal of restoring health to patients. However, there may be mismatches in terms of the health professional and his/her organisational goals. For example, if a person thrives on risk-taking, he/she may not fit well within the risk-averse environment that is necessary to ensure the delivery of a consistently high-quality service. A person with high security needs may not perform well in an environment that is characterised by short-term contract and acting posts.

Motivation

Motivation is intrinsically linked with needs and values. Maslow's work on motivation identifies a hierarchy of needs from basic biological needs to basic comfort through to self-actualisation. Hertzberg, famous for his two-factor theory, claimed that needs could be categorised as hygiene factors (pay, quality of supervision, fringe benefits and so on) and motivator factors (autonomy, recognition, opportunity to fulfill personal goals and so on). The absence of hygiene factors may result in dissatisfaction, whereas the presence of motivator factors is necessary for job satisfaction. In chapter 2 we discussed the influence of Argyris' and McGregor's theories on motivation. Attending to the motivation of employees is therefore likely to involve finding appropriate ways of enriching their jobs through greater autonomy, recognition and involvement in decision making. Some health services managers hold the view that it is difficult to motivate employees in the public service where there is very limited discretion on pay and reward. However, providing autonomy and involvement in decision-making is perhaps of equal, if not more, importance to health professionals, who, through their education and training, are led to expect that their opinions will be valued and that they will be expected to practice with a significant amount of autonomy.

Individual and Organisational Performance

Individual, group and organisational performance represent the output of the organisation. In the health services this is clearly the service delivered. Measurement of performance should therefore include throughput of patients, patient satisfaction, quality (as measured by health and social gain) and efficiency in terms of resource utilisation. In many instances performance measurement in healthcare is not yet sophisticated enough to take account of all of these measures and tends to focus for the most part on throughput.

A useful approach to measuring performance is the use of the balanced scorecard. The balanced scorecard is a customer-based planning and process improvement system aimed at focusing and driving an organisation's change process (Chow et al. 1998). It focuses on translating strategy into a set of financial and non-financial performance measures thus providing feedback to guide the improvement process. The details of the measures on the scorecard will vary from one organisation to another, but typically a scorecard would include at least the following four components:

- *Customer perspective*: How do customers see us?
- *Internal business perspective*: What do we need to excel on?
- *Innovation and learning*: Can we continue to improve and provide a better service?
- *Financial perspective*: How do our funders perceive our financial performance?

Chow et al. (1998), in exploring the application of the balanced scorecard to healthcare organisations, interviewed top-level administrators (e.g. hospital CEOs) and heads of laboratory services who agreed that the scorecard was valuable in measuring performance in the healthcare sector. By involving staff at all levels and all disciplines in the scorecard development process, "the organisation can ensure full and open communication of needs, concerns and ideas, increased understanding of needed actions, as well as acceptance and dedication to a shared set of goals" (1998: 278).

Kaplan and Norton (1996), who developed the balanced scorecard, provide three guidelines to help organisations select appropriate measures:

1. The performance measures selected should be positively related to the degree of attainment of the related goal, i.e. the measure should increase as the attainment of the goal increases.
2. Not all the performance measures should be focused on outcomes. Performance drivers should also be included as leading indicators: for example, the number of patients discharged could be an outcome measure and bed capacity might be an associated performance driver.
3. The number of performance measures should not be too great as a multitude of measures can cause the organisation to lose its focus and become disillusioned if progress is not made on the majority of measures.

CONCLUSIONS

The central message from the Burke-Litwin Model is that the transformational factors in the top half are the ones that drive and enable change. So planned change should follow the flow from top to bottom or from external environment to performance. This is congruent with open-systems theory, in that the external environment and the forces in the top half have more weight in making change happen. We know from experience that this is not always followed. In many instances change is enacted through a redesign of the organisation's structure, only to find a year later that while the boxes have changed, performance has not.

Case 4.2 The Restructuring of the Mid-Eastern Health Board

Two pieces of legislation were enacted in 1996 and 1997 that had major implications for the Irish health system. The Health Amendment Act clarified accountability of CEOs in relation to their health boards and the Freedom of Information Act gave every person the right to access information pertaining to him/her and the right to documentation relating to any decision taken by a public body. This meant that health boards had to be much more transparent in their decision making and that decisions had to be based on evidence and sound logic.

The Mid-Eastern Health Board in response to the enactment of the Health Amendment Act and in preparation for the Freedom of Information Act decided it needed to re-design its organisation and create clarity around the purpose of the organisation and who did what in order to achieve this purpose.

Phase one of this change process began with the CEO inviting a management consultant to work with the management team to develop a structure that would create a "strong culture of responsibility and accountability". The consultant met with each member of the management team individually to collect data about each person's current role and responsibilities, as well as their perceptions about accountability within the organisation. He then spent a half-day with the CEO in a private meeting after which he produced a draft structure for the CEO's consideration. The CEO discussed the structure with his deputy CEO who agreed that it was a major improvement on the existing structure. This was communicated back to the consultant who then arranged a management team "away day" to introduce the new structure to the rest of the management team and discuss the changes in their areas of responsibility. The essence of the new structure was a change from three programmes of care, i.e. community care, hospital care and special care (encompassing mental health and disabilities) to two geographical programmes integrating all three in each programme under the direction of an assistant CEO, with a third assistant CEO for strategy development. Each of the assistant CEOs (formerly "programme managers") was charged with explaining the new structure to those staff who would report to him/her within the geographical area. The CEO was to work closely with the assistant responsible for strategy development whose first task was to develop a five-year strategic plan for the Mid-Eastern Health Board.

Phase two of the change project began one month after phase one with the management team developing terms of reference and inviting tenders from consultancies for the mapping of existing policies and procedures for all aspects of the organisation. It was envisaged that this

cont/d

process would take a year. The consultancy firm who won the contract had a good reputation and a track record in re-designing large manufacturing companies. Although they had experience of working with some voluntary health organisations, they had not previously worked with a large healthcare organisation. They had recently recruited two consultants who had "extensive experience consulting to the NHS in the UK" and assured the CEO that these "experts" would "front the project".

The project got off to a good start and a team of four consultants worked their way methodically through the specialties and departments of the health board identifying a pilot hospital and a pilot community area on which to base policy and procedure manuals that would then be adopted by all similar specialties in the other geographical areas across the health board. They worked mainly by consulting existing documents, interviewing a random selection of middle managers and conducting some observations in the various locations. Apart from a few minor hiccups, such as one surgeon refusing them access to his wards, and a heated meeting between ward managers and the hospital managers where the ward managers accused the consultants of "spying" on them and "making patients uneasy", the work progressed according to plan. Eighteen months after the start date the health board launched its complete set of policy and procedure manuals for the entire organisation. The consultants were praised for their work and their contract ended.

Exactly eight months after this launch a letter arrived on the CEOs desk marked "strictly private and confidential". It was a letter from Mrs Greene, a former patient who complained that she had been admitted to her local hospital for an angiogram and was subsequently transferred to the hospital 30 miles away for further tests. After two days in this hospital, her doctor arrived on the ward with a woman who wanted to "have a chat with her" as her doctor explained. During the course of this "chat" the woman revealed that she was a psychiatrist.

Mrs Greene was very angry and left the hospital. When she calmed down she returned to make a complaint. She asked to see her doctor, but was told he had completed his training and was now working in Dublin. She then asked to see the psychiatrist's boss, but nobody seemed to know who her boss was. The letter went on to say that she did not consider herself to be suffering from any mental problems and would like an explanation or answer to the following:

- Why she had to talk to a psychiatrist.
- Why this meeting was arranged without her permission. and
- Why nobody on the ward seemed to know who this psychiatrist's boss was.

cont/d

Questions

1. Assuming the facts of Mrs Greene's letter are correct, what are your main concerns about responsibility and accountability in the Mid-Eastern Health Board?

2. Using the transformational and transactional variables of the Burke-Litwin model, examine the change process in the Mid-Eastern Health Board and re-design the process to ensure that letters from future "Mrs Greenes" do not become a frequent occurrence in the Mid-Eastern Health Board.

Clinical Inquiry Exercise 4.1

Identify a change that has recently been implemented in your organisation.

1. Use the Burke-Litwin model to identify how the change was initiated:
   a. Through transformational or transactional factors?
   b. Through which specific factors?

2. What impact is this change likely to have on the whole organisation in the longer term?

3. Does the Burke-Litwin model support your thinking on the impact of the change?

CHAPTER 5

Organisational Levels and Interlevel Dynamics

In the previous chapter we explored the notion of organisations as open and recursive systems. We introduced the Burke-Litwin model as a systems framework that describes and shows how transformational and transactional factors can be understood and used to construct and implement organisation change. Another way of seeing organisations as systems is through levels of analysis and aggregation. By levels of analysis we mean the individual level, the team or group level, the inter-group level and the organisational level. Several essential points need to be made about the concept and usage of the term "levels".

To begin with, the notion of levels must be distinguished from that of hierarchy. Hierarchy refers to position on a chain of command in an organisation, such as staff nurse, ward manager, divisional nurse manager and director of nursing. The less common use of organisational levels as a construct in organisational behaviour, however, describes levels of complexity. In biological systems, levels refer to levels of complexity, such as cell, organ, organism, group, organisation and society. They are ordered in a hierarchy of increasing complexity in that a system is composed of interrelated subsystems in a hierarchical order, i.e. organs are composed of cells, organisms are composed of organs and so on. In the health services an example from primary care is the social worker operating at the individual level in his/her clinical practice; the social work team (to which the social worker belongs) is the group level; the inter-group level might be the care groups, i.e. child care group and elderly care group consisting of several different professional groups; and the organisational level might be the community care team for the particular geographical area.

Levels of aggregation – individual, group, inter-group and organisation – are frequently used as frameworks for understanding organisational processes. Typically they are used to catalogue particular dynamics and interventions within OD efforts, i.e. career interventions at the individual level, team-building interventions at the group level and so on. Rarely is there any explicit discussion of how events on one level affect the dynamics of other levels. Yet in OD work experiences, it is clear that a triggering event in an organisation's external environment sets off a reformulation of strategy that can have consequent implications for the work of the organisation's teams and can affect how individual members view their membership of the organisation. Such examples require that organisational levels be understood less in static terms and that interlevel dynamics be constructed into OD theory and practice. One particular framework of organisational levels attempts to meet these issues and articulate an OD framework that acknowledges how large system change is an interlevel process.

FOUR LEVELS OF ORGANISATION BEHAVIOUR

Rashford and Coghlan (1994) present levels in terms of how people participate in organisations and link them to provide a useful tool for managers, consultants and teachers of organisation behaviour. Their framework describes four levels of participation or involvement in organisations (Table 5.1). These levels can be viewed as degrees of participation, or as degrees of complexity, depending on whether one approaches the question from the point of the view of the individual moving towards the organisation to participate or the part of the organisation viewing the commitment of individuals.

Table 5.1 Tasks at Each of the Four Organisational Levels

	LEVEL	TASK
1.	Individual	Bonding
2.	Face-to-Face-Team	Creating a functioning team
3.	Interdepartmental Group	Coordination
4.	Organisation	Adaptation

In the Rashford and Coghlan framework, the least complex approach, from the point of view of the individual, is the *bonding* relationship that the individual has with the organisation. This involves utilisation of membership and participation in the organisation in order to meet personal life goals (Level I). The more complex approach to participation exists in establishing *effective working relationships in a face-to-face team* (Level II). An even more complex involvement exists in terms of the interdepartmental group or divisional type of interface where teams must be *coordinated* in order to achieve complex tasks and maintain a balance of power among competing political interest groups (Level III). Finally, the most complex, from the point of view of the individual, is the relationship of the total organisation to its external environment in which other organisations are individual competitors, competing for scarce resources to produce similar products or services. The key task for any organisation is its ability to *adapt* to environmental forces driving for change (Level IV).

As an example in the health services environment, take a surgeon who works in a hospital because he/she has a personal goal to be a professional and to help people by performing procedures that save lives. At level II the surgeon needs to work with the surgical team, i.e. nurses, anaesthetists and so on, in order to perform these procedures. At level III the surgical team to which this doctor belongs needs to coordinate with other hospital departments – for example X-Ray, physiotherapy, occupational therapy – for after-care. At level IV there may be a requirement to comply with hospital policy on bed occupancy rates or day surgery initiatives and Department of Health and Children directives on waiting-list initiatives, which may impact on the work of the team and the individual doctor.

From management's perspective, the core issue is one of participation. The most basic participation is to get a person committed to the goals, values and culture of the organisation. The second level of participation is to establish good, working face-to-face relationships in functional teams. The third level of participation is the interdepartmental group or divisional level in which complex management information and data systems must be used to extend the knowledge and coordinate the functions of complex working divisions or service units. Finally, the most complex of all is the unified effort of all participants in an organisation towards the end of making the organisation work and achieve its goals, which can range from functionality to profitability to client-centredness to growth-orientation. In a hospital environment it is the unified effort of all that makes possible the diagnosis, treatment and care of patients that are referred from primary care. The construct of organisational levels forms a conceptual framework of different types of participation and involvement whereby many of the issues that arise in organisations can be understood and diagnosed.

Rashford and Coghlan (1994) distinguish task and interpersonal issues in terms of content, process and premise (Table 5.2). *Task content* refers to *what* the organisation, interdepartmental group, team or individual is intending to do: its mission and the tasks to be done (e.g. performing a surgical procedure such as a hip replacement). *Task process* refers to *how* the organisation, interdepartmental group, team or individual engages in defining the mission, setting goals, completing tasks, reviewing progress and so on (e.g. the steps that are followed such as assessment, admission, pre-operative care, procedure and recovery). *Task premise* refers to regular patterns that have been formed around critical task issues, such as, defining mission, selecting, setting and accomplishing goals, and problem-solving (admission and pre-op come before theatre). These patterns become taken for granted and viewed as basic assumptions, and so constitute the organisation's culture (Schein, 1999a).

Table 5.2 Template for Observation and Intervention

	TASK	RELATIONAL
CONTENT	*What* is done or intended	Roles people perform and play
PROCESS	*How* it is done	How people work together
PREMISE	Unquestioned patterns of task accomplishment	Recurrent interpersonal relationships and roles

Relational content refers to the particular roles the members of an organisation play with regard to other members – supporting, controlling, manipulating (e.g. the theatre nurse supports the surgeon). *Relational process* overlaps somewhat with relational content and focuses more on what is happening in the organisation, the interdepartmental group or team: how people work or do not work together and so on (to perform the operation, assistance is required from the anaesthetist, the theatre sister, the porter, the recovery team etc.). *Relational premise* refers to the basic assumptions governing how authority and peer relationships are defined, how thoughts and feelings are expressed, how influence is exercised and how crises are dealt with (e.g. a senior nurse deferring to a junior doctor, even though the nurse has more competence and expertise, as the junior doctor has only recently rotated into the speciality). This six-box framework provides a useful template for observing and for intervening.

Level I: Individual

Individuals within organisations have life-tasks, needs and wishes that extend far beyond their participation in any given work setting. Each individual person struggles to find unique and personalised satisfactions in this regard as they move through their adult life cycle and attempt to create a meaningful balance between their bio-social, work and family cycles (Schein, 1978). Management's perspective at the same point, however, is that individuals somehow belong to the organisation in an appropriate psychological contract. When the tasks at this level are reasonably and adequately met, individuals can allow the organisation and its goals to be a source of personal goal motivation. Individuals will still retain their own individuality while "belonging" to the organisation.

In contrast, it is the function of management to create the conditions whereby each individual is motivated so as to enhance individuals' growth and effectiveness. Therefore, management's ideal goal is to create a matching process in which people are able and encouraged to become involved, and find that the work situation develops them as human beings while the organisation benefits from such an involvement (Schein, 1978, 1993). For example, a nurse who is interested and experienced in nurse education and development, if freed from her clinical duties, could contribute to the development of many nurses in the organisation. This will result in personal satisfaction for this nurse, but also better performance for the organisation by those who have been the recipients of the training and development initiatives. Not all individuals relate to management's goals in this regard; some prefer to define their relationship to the organisation in political and adversarial terms, with the core issues at stake being power and control (Fox, 1985; Bolman and Deal, 1999).

There is an inevitable tension in this matching process (Argyris, 1990a; Schein, 1978). Individuals attempt to be themselves, bringing unique aspects of themselves to the organisation and, at the same time, adapting to organisational requirements and norms, as in, for example, the tension between providing the best quality care to individual patients against a health board's need to be resource efficient. One common difficulty here is that the plurality of views and theories-in-use as to how people are motivated produce contradictory approaches and undermine the growth process (McGregor, 1960; Schein, 1980). The manager who thinks that motivation is external and applied by coercion is in sharp contrast to the manager who thinks that motivation comes from within the person. The critical need is for managers to reflect on how different people might be motivated in diverse and changing situations, e.g. highly trained staff who work in stressful A&E situations and administrative staff whose working situation is more stable and predictable. The more ownership and awareness that individuals have of their lives, the more capable they are of contributing their unique aspects which are so necessary for organisations to change and develop.

Table 5.3 Focus of Observation and Intervention on Level I

	TASK	RELATIONAL
CONTENT	Job description, Role description and goal-setting	Career path
PROCESS	Job design, Performance review	Career interview
PREMISE	Managerial assumptions about work and work motivation	Psychological contract
OUTCOME	BONDING	

Table 5.3 applies the template to the individual level. The task issues on the individual level are the issues around job description, role description and goal setting (task content), performance review and job design (task process), and the managerial assumptions around work and work motivation (task premise). The relational issues are the individual's career path (relational content) and the career interview through which the career path is negotiated (relational process). These are supported or undermined by the psychological contract about organisations and the individual skills desired (relational premise).

Organisational change typically means that individual employees have to change too. Individuals may be required to change what they do or how they do it. It may be required of them to change their attitudes towards their work or some particular aspect of it. A consequence of this may be that an individual's sense of bonding to the changed or changing organisation may be altered, either positively or negatively. For example, if a community care area devolves budgets to heads of departments, a head occupational therapist will have to embrace budget management as part of his/her job. This may result in the occupational therapist feeling differently about the organisation, perhaps believing that it is no longer a caring organisation but one concerned primarily with finances.

An organisational change if not well-managed may result in individuals feeling demotivated and alienated, and exhibiting defensive behaviour. OD practitioners may work with individuals' negative perception of the change, which may be located in a particular individual's personality or in how the change is introduced and managed. The change process may also suggest that it would be useful for the OD practitioner to work at facilitating individuals to identify and evaluate the dynamics of the life-cycle, the work-cycle and the family-cycle, and place them in juxtaposition so that they can locate their career issues in the context of their lives. Individuals can be facilitated to take ownership of their lives and careers, and adopt positive coping responses to the tasks facing them. Furthermore, work with these individuals aims towards empowering them to suggest, initiate and promote change in the organisation and reduce undesired stressful side effects. For example, the OD practitioner might work with the occupational therapist to show that the positive side is that he/she can make key decisions about what services to develop without having to go through numerous frustrating attempts to persuade a manager who does not have a full understanding of the occupational therapy service. At the same time, work with managers enables them to reflect on and restructure managerial assumptions and behaviour towards their subordinates and colleagues. OD practitioners in this situation are facilitating the individual employee and the manager to become more aware of their separate and mutual needs as persons within the organisation as well as the needs of the organisation. As organisational change involves individual and personal change, attention to the individual in the context of the wider systemic change is critical for the success of the change process.

Level II: Face-to-Face Team

From the individual's perspective, entry into the work activity involves interfacing with other persons in clearly defined units. Face-to-face teams are typically formal groups and defined in terms of: face-to-face interaction, common objectives, psychological awareness of other members and self-definition as a team, with boundaries between members and non-members clearly defined. The team level is a more complex level than the individual level because of the increased number of participants and interactions. Teams are parts of a wider system in organisations and some of the dysfunctional issues that arise within the team may originate beyond the team in its technological and political interface with other teams. Problems that arise between teams are considered at Level III.

From the managerial perspective, any individual's task within the face-to-face team is to contribute to the collective ventures of the team. Management requires the team to be efficient and cooperative in its output towards the overall organisational task. Effective team functioning requires the team to be successful in accomplishing its tasks and skilled in learning from its experience in building and maintaining working relationships.

Table 5.4 Focus of Observation and Intervention on Level II

	TASK	RELATIONAL
CONTENT	Set and achieve team goals	Team roles
PROCESS	Allocation of work to team members	Team processes
PREMISE	Standard operating procedures	Recurrent interpersonal relationships and roles
OUTCOME	CREATING A FUNCTIONING TEAM WHICH IS PRODUCTIVE	

Table 5.4 applies the template to the team level. The task issues for the face-to-face team are setting and achieving objectives (task content) and allocating the work to the members (task process), while the relational issues are how the members work together (relational content) and the team process (relational process). In health organisations, understanding the relational content of teams and groups may be helpful in mapping

how different disciplines may contribute to a multi-disciplinary team (Ovretveit, 1993; Barker and Barker, 1994) For example, multi-disciplinary teams comprising consultants, nurses and administration need to have an understanding of the perspectives of each professional group in order to minimise perceptions of political posturing and to develop the possibilities of reaching consensus and improving the service. Relational content also refers to the styles of working in a group that individual team members bring to the teams.

Belbin (1981) identifies the following roles that he judges to be essential if a team is to be effective: specialist, completer, implementer, teamworker, monitor, evaluator, shaper, coordinator, resource investigator and plant. Some of these roles emphasise the creation of vision in a team's work, others focus on task accomplishment, while others attend to team issues. Each of these roles plays a key part in enabling a team to deal with complex issues. Other approaches, such as the Myers-Briggs Type Indicator (a scale based on Jung's theory of psychological types that is concerned with the valuable differences in people that result from where they like to focus their attention, the way they like to take in information, the way they like to decide and the kind of lifestyle they adopt), are also useful. An OD practitioner can help the members of the team identify the composite strengths of the mix of personality types and styles, and feel less anxious about working together in the face of different styles or an imbalance of styles.

The premise of the task and relational issues refers to the standard operating procedures and the recurring interpersonal relationships and roles that are operative but unstated and have become taken for granted. A team may have a procedure that is unstated and unquestioned whereby critical issues are never resolved because an analysis of causes is never done. A team may have an unstated premise of "peace at all costs" so the norm is not to confront or disagree, or there may be a pattern that certain members of a team have higher status than others and are listened to more than others (relational premise).

It is critical for face-to-face teams to develop the appropriate skills of self-reflection and correcting their own dysfunctions. Such skills typically constitute the definition of successful teams. Level II dysfunctions occur when assumptions, attitudes and behaviour of team members towards one another and the team's effort frustrate the team's performance (Wheelan, 1999). Generally, the discovery of negative information is not valued in many organisations as people then tend to fail to confront one another or else confront one another out of learned patterns of inference, attribution and the placing of blame (Argyris 1990b). Behaviours such as blaming, withholding information, inappropriate team leader style, misplaced competition, sexism, racism and lack of trust can negatively influence the team members' capacity to work well together and also inhibit team development. Furthermore, within any given team the interaction skills of task achievement and maintenance function may not be equally developed.

The change agenda in an organisation typically affects the work of teams. Teams may set new goals and targets. They may have to work differently. For example, the 'Clinicians in Management' initiative changed the structure of hospitals to group multi-disciplinary teams around specialties such as elderly care, cardiac care and so on. The purpose of this re-structuring was to encourage teams to work differently and to share expertise with other professionals working in similar clinical areas. The new goal was more integrated patient care.

OD has long focused on the pivotal role of groups in organisational change. The process of organisational change typically involves the change agenda being assessed and responded to by the permanent working teams in the organisation's structure and by the involvement of temporary committees, task forces or action learning sets in solving problems, creating policy or generating commitment. Level II processes may occur in the permanent teams that are the basis of the structures of most organisations. In this context the long-term relationships among the members and the patterns of interaction that have become taken for granted and have become largely unnoticed can be a significant area of focus and intervention for the OD practitioner. In the context of temporary groups, such as task forces, *ad hoc* committees and action learning sets, the OD practitioner, as well as attending to issues of task achievement and interpersonal dynamics, should also attend to how the task force relates to and is integrated into the structure and culture of the organisation. If a team works in isolation from the organisation with no permeability between it and the other parts of the organisation, it will be difficult to integrate the results.

For example, a task force to develop a customer relations strategy for the organisation must work with all levels and inform staff as the work progresses if it is to succeed in implementing the strategy further down the line. Equally, a design task force working on the plans for a new wing of the hospital must consult with the people who will work in this space, otherwise they may find they have overlooked some vital components (as happened recently when nursing staff moved into a newly opened ward and found that the beds were too close together to allow them to work effectively). One important aspect of the OD practitioner's work at this second level is to enable a team (whether a permanent team or a temporary task force) to build its team skills (Wheelan, 1999).

Level III: Interdepartmental Group

This third level can be made up of any number of face-to-face working teams, units or services that must function together to accomplish an interdepartmental service delivery purpose. This interdepartmental group level needs to have critical information that passes beyond the boundaries of individual teams in order to implement programmes and projects at a range beyond their direct contact. In large organisations where size and distance dissolve immediate personal relationships, it is imperative that this third level functions well. From management's standpoint, the team's task within the overall group is to perform effectively in its own right, while at the same time have a clearly defined commitment to the interdepartmental group. When this third level is working effectively, people in the interdepartmental group are capable of obtaining information and converting it into decision processes, enabling the implementation of complex programmes or operations. Hence the task at this level is to map the flow of information and partially completed work from one team to another. In hospital care, the transfer of information and the process of patient care, which requires work by admissions, ward and theatre respectively, and involves X Ray, physiotherapy and catering, illustrate the complexity of coordination at this level.

The structure of industrial relations occurs at this level. While the overall strategy of industrial relations takes place at national level, good relations between management and unions, and between unions themselves, in the concrete exercise of partnership at the local level is a feature of effective working of Level III (Gunnigle, McMahon and Fitzgerald, 1999; *National Framework Agreement, 2000*; D'Art and Turner, 2002).

Table 5.5 Focus of Observation and Intervention on Level III

	TASK	RELATIONAL
CONTENT	Division of organisational functions Division of resources Structure of management information systems	Resource exchange Quality of information Timely information Collective bargaining outcomes
PROCESS	Determination of compatibility Determination of input/output Determination of specialties or professional field to the organization	Decision support systems PERT, internal mapping Allocation of resources to fit input/output Collective bargaining
PREMISE	Assumptions and sharing of information and resources	Sub-cultures (functional areas, specialisations and professions)
OUTCOME	COORDINATION	

Table 5.5 applies the template to the interdepartmental group level. The task issues at this third level are the division of organisational functions and resources, and the structure of the information system to support the differentiation. Task process refers to how these functions are compatible and how the work flows from one function to another. Relational issues focus on the quality and timeliness of information exchange, collective bargaining outcomes (relational content), and decision-support systems and the collective-bargaining process (relational process). Task and relational premise at this level refers to assumptions about information sharing and resource allocation arising from sub-cultures within and between functions.

The process of performing a complex function and making an appropriate distribution of scarce resources, such as personnel and money, are the key ventures of the interdepartmental group level. It is a highly political situation in which the inbuilt structural conflicts of multiple interest parties need to be resolved. As a group, this diversified mass of differing functions and interests must negotiate an outcome that adequately reflects the balance of power and a distribution of resources among competing coalitions. Essential elements in Level III dynamics centre on issues of power and on how power is exercised in the allocation of resources and the accessibility of information.

From management's view the technical issues at this level require an ability to locate dysfunctions. Dysfunctions occur in the flow of transferring information and partially completed work or services from one team to another. The entire process must be viewed, understood and successfully handled in order to produce the product or service. Because of a huge number of individuals engaged in particular activities in a large organisation, this process is often difficult to see. The interdepartmental group's process then must focus on becoming a functioning work unit to build on successes and learn from mistakes. Difficulties also arise at this level due to the lack of reflective and corrective skills. Discovery of negative information is difficult because it is often hidden in the interfaces between one team and another.

The interdepartmental group is critical in an organisational change. As resources are re-allocated and technology and advanced information systems alter access to the flow of information, teams are required to communicate more effectively across functions and departments. Such a process may involve integral cultural change (Schein, 1999a). OD practitioners can enable the interdepartmental group to locate problems through the use of internal mapping. Internal mapping utilises a process whereby individual heads of work units or team leaders are facilitated to plot the work flow through their section, and to do this in such a way that from the beginning of a work process to its finish, all the intermediate links between different functioning teams are plotted and all the members of the group then have a chance to *jointly* take ownership of all the dysfunctional areas and proceed to work in small task forces in order to remedy the dysfunctions.

OD practitioners may also facilitate situations in which inter-team tensions require resolution. This can be done by providing a safe environment in which inter-functional relations can be examined and discussed in a manner that enables protagonists to actively listen to one another and come to understand experiences and perspectives of teams other than their own. In a similar vein industrial relations mediation or facilitation may serve to bring representatives together to address emergent problems and issues and resolve them in accordance with national agreements and agreed procedures.

Another important intervention at this level is the use of large group processes (Bunker and Alban, 1997; Coghlan, 1998), such as "search/future search conferences" (Weisbord and Janoff, 1995; Emery and Purser, 1996;), "whole scale change" (Dannemiller, 2000) and "open space" (Owen, 1997) where organisational members from all functional and geographical areas come together for a number of days and:

- Review the past.
- Explore the present.
- Create an ideal future scenario.
- Identify common ground.
- Make action plans.

The significance of these approaches is that they enable the whole system to engage in strategic thinking and planning in an integrated manner within a defined period of time in a way that is dialogical, participative, draws on metaphoric approaches as well as rational ones and builds ownership of strategy and change agendas.

Level III is the level that requires most attention from OD in the Irish health system. With the restructuring of community care to care groups and the devolving of management in hospitals to directorates/integrated management units, matrix-type structures are becoming increasingly common. A matrix structure demands that an individual in that matrix reports to more than one manager. This scenario can create tensions in the organisation that will affect performance if they are not addressed. Figure 5.1 shows a typical matrix structure for a care group for the elderly. In this type of structure the public health nurse may find herself torn by the demands of the director of public health nursing and the director of services for the elderly. Managing and reducing this tension requires shared goals and a good working relationship between the care of the elderly planning team and the public health nursing team. The health system experiences continuing difficulties in moving between structures, whether this be in the community services or in the hospital services. This difficulty seems to arise from an over-focusing on getting the structures right and a lack of attention to the support necessary to build new relationships and encourage teams to work differently. As Mintzberg (1997: 18) points out "if even a fraction of the efforts that are put into moving positions around on charts went into moving people around on floors, there might be an awful lot more collaborative activities in hospitals".

Figure 5.1 Services for the Elderly – Matrix Structure

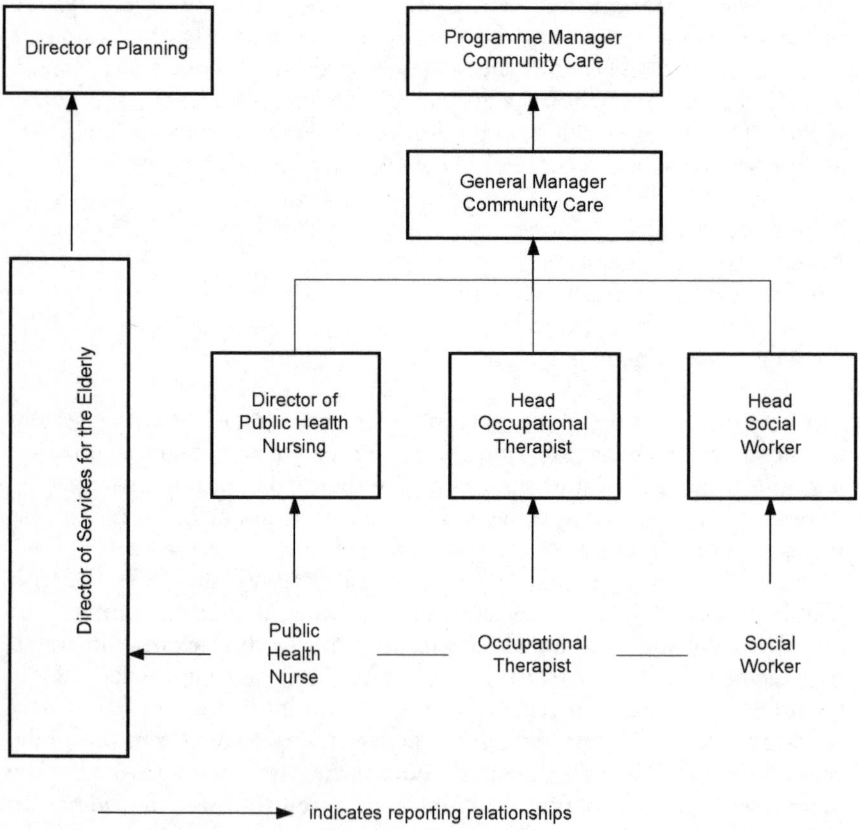

indicates reporting relationships

Level IV: Organisation

The fourth level relates to the organisational goals, policy and strategy level, which constitutes the fusion of all three levels together to form a working, cohesive organisation that provides a service according to its mission. The organisation's tasks are to have a unified corporate identity and to exist in a competitive environment. Consequently, an organisation needs to be capable of reflecting on its own strengths and weaknesses, as well as engaging in proactive relationships to determine and deal with the opportunities and threats from the external environment. The assessment of strengths, weaknesses, opportunities and threats results in a selection process that establishes programmes and services. These procedures aim at accomplishing the goals of the organisation and adapting to external environmental demands. An awareness of the cultural assumptions which underlie any organisation's policies, strategies, structures and behaviours contributes to the successful completion of the tasks at this level.

Table 5.6 Focus of Observation and Intervention on Level IV

	TASK	RELATIONAL
CONTENT	Survival and profitability Quality of service delivery Attainment of mission Sense of organisational worth	Stakeholder service
PROCESS	Strategic planning and management	Management of change Organisational learning
PREMISE	Organisational self-image	Organisational environmental image
OUTCOME	ADAPTATION	

Table 5.6 applies the template to the organisation level. The separation of task and relational issues under the headings of content, process and premise at this level enables managers and OD practitioners distinguish issues for the purposes of diagnosis and intervention. A list of such issues typically includes: survival, quality of service delivery, profitability, attainment of mission, sense of organisational worth (task content), open system planning, strategic planning and management (task process), competitive advantage, stakeholder service (relational content), organisational adaptation and learning, and the management of change (relational process). In the past five years healthcare organisations in this country have given a great deal of attention to strategic planning, establishing goals, mission and strategy for organisations. However, for the most part, the relational aspects have not received the same attention as the task aspects. This has resulted in systems with limited capacity for change.

OD practitioners work with senior managers on developing an appropriate approach to strategy, deciding who should be involved in the processes of planning, developing options and implementation, how the process could work most effectively and what additional expert external help could be utilised. OD practitioners can help the members of an organisation clarify their core mission, map the internal and external constituencies that make demands on the organisation and its strategic choices, and assess the strengths, weaknesses, opportunities and threats both externally and internally. For example, a methodology such as open systems planning can be usefully utilised. Open systems planning comprises elements of identifying key environmental stakeholders and analysing the demands they are currently making on the organisation, the projected demands they will make, the current responses to those demands, creation of a desired future and action planning. OD practitioners can also help members of an organisation question the assumptions underlying the management and implementation of planning processes and take steps to deal with those issues which, if not attended to, would ultimately lead to failure (Argyris, 1985).

Inter-Organisational Networks
A dynamic within the organisation level is the increasing development of participation in inter-organisational networks, such as the partnerships between universities and hospitals regarding the education of health professionals.

The dynamics of inter-organisational networks in many ways are not dissimilar to those at the interdepartmental group level. They involve relating and working with other systems that have different perspectives, priorities, goals, traditions and ways of working. It is akin to diplomatic relationships with foreign countries and cultures. The challenge for those who engage in face-to-face interaction with members of other systems on behalf of their own system is to create and build common ground that enhances each participating system, rather than attempts to make gains at the expense of the others. Hence the development of trust interpersonally, between the representatives of the systems initially, and inter-organisationally is essential.

Rashford and Coghlan's (1994) framework of four organisational levels encompasses the literature on the individual-organisation relationship, team dynamics, inter-team relationships, management information and decision support systems, organisational strategic planning and management, and organisational change and development. Level I utilises the issues in individual–organisational relationships, human resource management and career dynamics; Level II team dynamics; Level III inter-team dynamics, industrial relations and management decision support systems, and Level IV strategic planning and management, and organisational change and development. The Rashford and Coghlan framework attempts to integrate macro issues (strategy, organisational change and development, competitive survival, management information systems and technology) and micro issues (individual bonding, motivation, individual psychology and group dynamics) into a single concept. It complements the Burke-Litwin model by focusing on how the people in the organisation relate to the transformational and transactional factors.

INTERLEVEL DYNAMICS

There is an essential interlevel element in that each level has a dynamic relationship with each of the others. This relationship is grounded in systems dynamics, whereby the relationship each of the four levels has with the other three is systemic, with feedback loops forming a complex pattern of relationships. Dysfunctions at any of the four levels can cause dysfunctions at any of the other three levels. An individual's level of stress can be expressed in dysfunctional behaviour in the team and affect a team's ability to function effectively, which in turn affects the individual's ability to cope and ultimately the bonding relationship with the organisation. If a team is not functioning effectively, it can limit the interdepartmental group's effectiveness, which may depend on the quality and timeliness of information, resources and partially completed work from that team. If the interdepartmental group's multiple activities are not coordinated, the organisation's ability to compete effectively may be affected. In systemic terms, each of the four levels affects each of the other three.

While the framework of organisational levels focuses on levels as a notion of complexity rather than a position on the hierarchy of command, positioning on a chain of command has an impact on the functioning of the four levels. When an individual has a problem, the higher he/she is on the hierarchy the greater the impact is on the organisation. The higher one is on the hierarchy or the more power a team has the greater the influence to bring about change. The inter-connectedness between positions on the hierarchy and levels of complexity exists in the role of the "key" individual. The key individual is a general term to connote those whose roles involve crossing boundaries from one subsystem to another (Ancona and Caldwell, 1988). A typical example of a key individual crossing sub-systems in a hospital setting is the bed manager. Team-leaders, supervisors, managers and administrators all cross the boundary from their area of responsibility to those of other functions or higher management. This constitutes crossing boundaries within the hierarchy. At the same time, these individuals are interacting in interlevel dynamics. They bring individual issues to a team, and team issues to the interdepartmental group. When an individual represents his/her own department to a broader function, he/she crosses from the team to the group level and the dynamic of that interaction may lead to a re-assessment of the individual level. Other interlevel interaction occurs in the "gatekeeping" role (Ancona and Caldwell, 1988), whereby new information is brought into the team from the external environment. New information, especially disconfirming information, may cause the individual to be rejected by the team. As will be discussed below, as the process of change moves between the four levels the persons who move the change between the levels are significant.

Organisational change is a multi-level activity as fundamental systemic change requires behavioural change on all four levels. This is not easy as interventions on one level may contradict interventions on other levels – an individual incentive scheme may work against teambuilding (for example, a performance management system that rewards individual achievement). It may also be that what is intended as multi-level change may not in fact be so – teambuilding for the top management team may not have an organisation-wide impact. The quality movement is an example of how interlevel dynamics are operative. Quality affects the work of individuals, teams and how teams and units interact and perform their own tasks in relation to one another. Any one of those can have an impact on any or each of the others. OD practitioners can use the construct of the four levels as a diagnostic framework by being aware of the issues occurring at each level and how one level affects another, and be able to work with individuals, teams and inter-team groups to evaluate the effect of one level on another. As we will see in the next chapter, the process of moving a change through an organisation – creating a vision of the changed state, planning interventions, building commitment and managing the transition – requires a systemic view of the complex inter-relationship and interdependence of the individual, the face-to-face team, the interdepartmental group and the organisation.

In this process of evaluating the impact of one level on another, OD practitioners must take notice of the systemic nature of the relationship between each of the levels, that is to say, to construct how the relationship between one level and another works in both directions (Figure 5.2). As discussed in the previous chapter, an individual's sense of alienation from the team in which she works, not only affects her participation in the team and the team's work, but also what happens in the team affects her sense of alienation. When relationships are viewed as systems, then there is no simple cause-and-effect linear chain. There is no direct line of blame. Each element in the system both causes and is caused by the other elements.

Viewing the organisation as a whole comprising the four interrelated and interdependent levels enables OD practitioners adopt a systemic approach to the consultation. As we indicated in chapter 4, methods from the Milan approach to family therapy – examining circularity, developing and testing hypotheses in order to establish links and patterns, to explore meanings and covert rules which hold situations in place – may be usefully adopted to help a client system understand the complexities of its

Figure 5.2 Systemic Interlevel Change

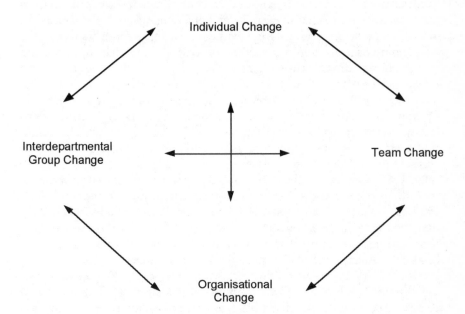

interlevel dynamics (Campbell, Draper and Huffington, 1991; Campbell, Coldicott and Kinsella, 1994; McCaughan and Palmer, 1994). Interlevel dynamics can also be viewed from a psycho-analytic perspective (Schneider, 1991). For OD practitioners who work from a psycho-analytic perspective, the psycho-analytic systems approach of the Tavistock Institute focuses on the psycho-dynamics of crossing boundaries from one level to another (Rice, 1990).

The Rashford and Coghlan (1994) framework of four organisational levels aims at such a task as it confronts the linkages between the levels. It attempts to articulate the dynamic inter-relationship between the individual's bonding to the organisation, the team's functioning, the interdepartmental group's coordination and the organisation's adaptation. OD practitioners are constantly dealing with the effects of one level on another, yet this interlevel reality as a focus for diagnosis and intervention is rarely given expression in the organisational change and development literature.

CONCLUSIONS

In this chapter we have presented a framework of organisational levels. The construct of organisational levels is essentially systemic and emphasises the dynamic inter-relationship between each of the four levels. The inter-relationship and interdependence of the four levels is highlighted in the context of systemic organisational change, whereby an organisation attempts to adapt to changing environmental demands, which necessitates a re-alignment of the interdepartmental group's coordination, the functioning of teams and the bonding process of individuals to a changed or changing organisation. The task of adaptation requires the interdepartmental group to re-configure its relationships – the re-allocation of resources, access to information, collective bargaining between management and unions, and inter-team politics. Each level has its own task or purpose – bonding on Level I, creating a functioning team on Level II, coordination on Level III and adaptation on Level IV – which requires the management of the fulfilment of each purpose and the inter-relationship between each purpose. Each level can be viewed in terms of its task and how the tasks of each level are affected in an organisational change. OD practitioners can use organisational levels as a framework for diagnosis and intervention by seeing a) how change is required *at* each level and intervening to help that happen and b) how what happens on each level affects each of the other levels and so intervening *between* the levels. We have provided illustrations of possible OD concerns and interventions (Table 5.7). These examples are illustrative and not intended to be comprehensive or exhaustive. Such a focus on interlevel dynamics is essential in order to understand and manage the change process in a complex organisation.

Table 5.7 Examples of OD Interventions at the Four Organisational Levels

LEVEL	Task at Each Level in the Context of a Changing Organisation	Examples of OD Interventions
I Individual	Bonding in the face of changing work, jobs, roles, career, organisational atmosphere, structures, culture...	Facilitating the management of resistance to change Work, job, role redesign Career counselling
II Team	Creating functioning, working teams in the permanent teams and temporary teams to deal with the change process	Facilitating task issues Facilitating interpersonal issues Teaching team skills
III Inter-departmental Group	Coordination of 1. cross-functional departments and interests, 2. information and resource exchange to meet the change issues	Interdepartmental cooperation and conflict management Mapping work flow Facilitating search conferences
IV Organisation	Adoption of the whole organisation to meet the driving forces for change and maintain quality service	Clarifying assumptions about the organisation and the environment Testing approaches to strategy Facilitating the formulation and implementation of strategy
Interlevel System	Systemic harmony	Exposing the feedback loops of how each level affects each of the others with respect to the change process

Case 5.1 Integrating Care

Catherine Collins is a 64-year-old lady who lives with her husband Jack in a small terraced house. Jack is 66 and suffers from arthritis. He had to stop driving 2 years ago because of this, and as Catherine never learnt to drive this has left Jack and Catherine without their own transport.

Three years ago Catherine started having problems with her hips. She had a lot of pain and seemed to be having difficulty walking. She also found that if she had to stand for any period of time the pain got worse. Jack persuaded Catherine to go to her G.P. She phoned to make an appointment with her G.P in the first week of January. When she arrived at the surgery for her appointment she was told that Dr Brady, her G.P., was still on his Christmas holidays, but his locum Dr Keane would see her. Catherine liked Dr Keane, a young female G.P who spent a long time talking to her. She explained to Catherine that as people get older they find the cold weather more difficult to cope with, and she recommended that Catherine go home and keep warm. She suggested to Catherine that she might come back to see Dr Brady in April if her pain did not "ease off" by then.

Catherine went home and struggled on. She turned up the heating, got a high stool for her kitchen so she could sit whilst cooking and washing dishes and tried not to complain too much, as she knew that Jack was also in a lot of pain with his arthritis. Her legs gradually got worse, but she dutifully waited until April before contacting Dr Brady.

In April, Dr Brady told Catherine that she might need an operation to cure her and referred her to Dr Nolan, the orthopaedic consultant at the local hospital. Three weeks later she received an appointment and took a taxi to the hospital. As this was Catherine's first appointment at the hospital, she wasn't sure if they would keep her in and do the operation or send her home again. She was very worried about this and didn't sleep very well the night before her appointment. The consultant told Catherine that she needed both hips replaced and as there was a long waiting list for this type of operation, she might not be called back for 10 months or more. Catherine went home very disappointed.

One year later, Catherine phoned the hospital to ask if they could send a nurse to help Jack get her in and out of bed, because she could no longer manage alone. The person she spoke to said that the hospital didn't send out nurses, and gave her the number of the Community Care office to contact. Catherine phoned the office and explained that she was Mr Nolan's patient and was having problems getting out of bed. The girl she spoke to explained to Catherine that she should contact Mr. Nolan who, as her consultant, has responsibility for any decisions relating to her care.

cont/d

Catherine phoned the hospital again and asked for Mr Nolan's clinic. She explained her problem to the secretary, who then asked her to hold on while she checked Catherine's place on the waiting list. She told Catherine that she would be called for operation next month and said Mr Nolan had asked if she could manage at home until then. Catherine was so delighted to hear she was finally going to have her operation that she said "yes" she could manage. She regretted this later that day when she saw the difficulty Jack was having trying to help her to get from the chair to the toilet. However, Catherine decided that the people in the hospital were so busy that she could not possibly bother them again.

Six weeks later, Catherine received a letter on Tuesday asking her to come in to hospital the following Monday. Catherine got herself ready, packed her clothes and booked a taxi for 7 a.m. on Monday morning. At 7 p.m. on Sunday evening Catherine received a call from the hospital to say that because an accident victim needed an emergency operation, her appointment had been cancelled.

Catherine received another phone call on Wednesday asking her to come in Thursday. She worried all Wednesday night that it would be cancelled again. Thankfully she was admitted on Thursday as planned. However, she did not have her operation until Monday, despite being wheeled down to the theatre twice. The first time the session ran way over schedule because of complications in a hernia operation. The second time there had been another emergency. Finally, Catherine was slotted in because of a spontaneous remission in an appendicitis case, an hour and a half before his operation was due.

Catherine was told her operation was successful and she was discharged from hospital ten days later. She suffered a lot of pain and stiffness during her subsequent weeks of recovery, but because of her experience trying to get help before going into hospital she did not know who to ask for help. She also thought the hospital might think her ungrateful if she phoned and asked for more help, as after all they had told her the operation was successful and as far as they were concerned she was cured. Catherine did not expect to feel so bad after the operation. She worried that maybe something had gone wrong and the hospital had missed it. Catherine did not want to give Jack the impression that the operation had not been successful, because he had been so hopeful that it would be the answer to all their problems. She kept her worries to herself. Catherine and Jack struggled on until eventually Catherine got back on her feet again.

Several months later Catherine ran into Dr Brady at her local supermarket. He asked her if she had heard anything from the hospital yet, and was very surprised to hear she'd already had her operation!

Questions

1. If the aim is to provide better continuity of care for Catherine, what

cont/d

needs to be addressed at levels I to IV to enable this continuity?
2. What interventions would you suggest and at what levels could these be targeted to best effect?

Clinical Inquiry Exercise 5.1

	Individual	Team	Interdepart-mental Group	Organisation
Individual				
Team				
Interdepartmental Group				
Organisation				

- Name a change issue with regard to an individual.
- Now work diagonally along the shaded boxes. How does one level have an impact on the others?
- Where would you put your energies to advance the progress of the change and heal dysfunctions?

Clinical Inquiry Exercise 5.2

1. Name a change issue that applies to the whole organisation.
2. Now work diagonally along the shaded boxes. How does one level have an impact on the others?
3. Develop strategies to implement change at each level.

PART III

ORGANISATION DEVELOPMENT IN ACTION

CHAPTER 6

Data in Action

In OD work action research entails systematically gathering data of whatever form on the nature of the particular issue, working with other participants at analysing the data and then taking action on the basis of that analysis (Cunningham, 1993; Waclawski and Church, 2002). In this chapter we explore some general themes around gathering data, making a diagnosis of an organisation and the role that formally collecting data plays in providing feedback to the organisation as the basis for further action.

Conventional research is based on vertical thinking in that a problem or issue is identified and broken down into more discrete parts until a problem that can be researched or a question that needs an answer is identified. Action research by contrast is based on lateral thinking, in that a problem or issue is identified and answers are found or questions generated by using ideas from other fields, looking at variables in other parts of the organisation, how variables interact with each other and so on. Lateral thinking, therefore, involves two aspects: the deliberate generation of alternative ways of looking at things and the challenging of assumptions (Cunningham, 1993). In research settings, this might involve defining the problem from a number of perspectives, using different theoretical frameworks to investigate a problem and having different and opposing viewpoints to solving the problem.

MULTIPLE REALITIES AND THE USE OF MULTIPLE PERSPECTIVES

One major development in OD has been the recognition that in many organisations there is little agreement among various organisational groups regarding the interpretations and evaluations of organisational events (Pettigrew, 1985; Brown and Covey, 1987; Ramirez and Bartunek, 1989). These different groups tend to have divergent perceptions of "shared" events. Such divergent perceptions have been termed "multiple realities" (Brown and Covey, 1987). They are particularly likely to exist in organisations such as healthcare organisations that have highly specialised disciplines and high status, role and goal differentiation (Strasser and Bateman, 1983). In settings containing multiple realities, groups operating from differing perceptions pursue their own goals, and conflict and political behaviours are inevitable (Greiner and Schein, 1988). Multiple realities are likely to lead to differing perceptions of the value of any particular intervention, a fact which must be taken account of in designing OD evaluations. Legge (1985) and Pettigrew (1985) suggest that multiple realities have implications for the assessment of OD. In these circumstances it is not sufficient to conduct "before and after" or "snapshot" evaluations of interventions. Instead it is necessary to track the process of the intervention using qualitative methodologies which enable the variety of different perceptions and reactions to be registered (Ramirez and Bartunek, 1989).

Many aspects of organisational life are difficult to define and as such it may be impossible to identify concepts for which there are accurate measures that will give a complete picture of the organisation. For example, we may want to know if poor practices exist in a clinical setting but cannot measure this by observing behaviour as the very presence of an observer would surely cause people to alter their behaviour. Thus we may have to make do with measures such as attitudes and perceptions or reported error rates. Each of these measures only partially describes the reality of the situation and as such could be described as biased.

In order to overcome such biases and the difficulties presented by multiple realities, generating data from a variety of perspectives and viewpoints is a developing tradition in the social sciences and has been described as multi-method or triangulation. The aim of these methods is to use qualitative and quantitative data together, as well as multiple levels of information and perspectives to provide different viewpoints on a research issue (Cunningham, 1993). The word triangulation has been defined as a combination of methodologies in the study of the same phenomenon and has been associated with practices in navigation and military strategy where multiple reference points are used to locate a ship's position.

There are several different types of triangulation:

- *Between methods*: using different methods to collect the same data: for example, using interviews and a survey instrument to gauge opinion on a new nurse-rostering system.
- *Within methods:* the use of multiple techniques within the same method: for example, using two different decision-making questionnaires to measure the level of involvement middle managers have in decision making.
- *Multiple frameworks or methods*: for example, combining qualitative and quantitative data to measure staff's understanding of organisational values, or combining data from staff nurses and from directors of nursing on the perceived organisational climate.
- *Multiple researchers*: having different observers or groups conducting

the research or analysing the data: for example, in researching resource allocation methods one might wish to get a health economist's perspective and a social scientist's perspective on the methods.

The underlying assumption in all triangulation is that weaknesses in one perspective, method or design can be strengthened by the counterbalancing influence of another.

Organisation development uses action research to help participants solve problems, identify solutions and put these into practice. This involves assuring that:

1. The relevant information for problem solving is available and understandable.
2. The information is capable of being utilised and manipulated by the system.
3. The cost of obtaining, understanding and using the data is not beyond the system's capacity.
4. The problem is solved and the decision implemented in such a way that it does not reoccur (i.e. an understanding of the contributory factors means that reoccurrence can be prevented).
5. The process of information use can be accomplished without damaging the implementation process (Argyris, 1970).

DATA-GATHERING APPROACHES

There are many approaches to gathering data that are useful in OD work. Here we will discuss the most commonly used approaches: surveys, interviews, focus groups, critical incidents, observation, rapid appraisal, delphi technique and nominal group technique.

Organisational Surveys in OD

A survey can be defined as any process used for asking people questions to gain information. This information can be attitudinal, factual, based on perceptions, beliefs or judgements. An organisational survey is "a systematic process of data collection designed to quantitatively measure specific aspects of organisational members' experience as they relate to work" (Church and Waclawski, 2001: 4). Organisational surveys are useful tools in OD. Indeed as we have seen one of the core roots in the development of OD is the pioneering survey work in organisations by Rensis Likert and his colleagues in Michigan. There are many useful guides to survey design and implementation that can be found in books on research. It is not our intention to reproduce these here but rather to discuss how surveys can be used in OD and how their use differs from their use in traditional research. There are multiple possible uses for surveys in OD work. Church and Waclawski (2001) identify the following significant categories of use:

- To understand and explore employee opinions, attitudes, values and beliefs.
- To provide a general or specific assessment of the behaviours and attributes inherent in employees' day-to-day work experience.
- To create baseline measures and use these for benchmarking various behaviours, processes and other aspects of organisations against either external or internal measures.
- To use the data for driving organisational change and development.

Waclawski and Church (2002) outline four ways in which the use of surveys in OD differs from the use in traditional research:

1. Building on what we explored in chapter 4, organisations are living systems that are part of and react to their external environment and have complex interrelationships and interdependences between internal factors, such as strategy, structure, culture, technology and so on. Surveys in OD work, therefore, are directed towards affecting or predicting organisational outcomes, such as performance.
2. Surveys in OD are model driven, that is they are based on specific or conceptual models that depict how an organisation functions.
3. Surveys in OD are action research oriented and are used as the basis for diagnosis. We will discuss diagnosis later in this chapter.
4. Surveys in OD are the springboard and instrument of intervention for action planning and change. The results of a survey point to what may be most important in a change project and are the basis for selecting appropriate interventions.

Interviews in OD

Interviews are very useful in OD. They provide an alternative perspective to that provided by surveys. Interviews are used for two purposes in OD (Waclawski and Church, 2002):

1. Interviews can be used for diagnostic purposes. OD practitioners can interview managers, team members and selected employees as to their views on what the key issues or main problems to be addressed are. These views provide OD practitioners with rich information as to how issues are perceived and this data can contribute to the diagnosis of the issues and act as the basis for action planning.
2. In OD, interviews are used to gather exploratory data used for three

primary purposes. The first is to obtain preliminary input for designing additional diagnostic tools. So, for example, interviews may indicate what questions might be asked in a survey. The second is that interviews may be used to follow up on data in more detail. This is where the interviews come after the survey and pick up on particular responses that might need further elaboration. The third purpose of exploratory interviews is in evaluation where, as a follow-up to an OD project, interviews are held to find out how the outcomes of the OD project are perceived.

The negative aspects of interviewing as a data-collection method is that it can be very resource intensive and time consuming.

Focus Groups in OD

An alternative method of collecting people's views is through a focus group, which is "a planned discussion designed to obtain perceptions on a defined area of interest in a permissive non-threatening environment" (Waclawski and Church, 2002: 115). Focus groups can be used for exploratory purposes and can be a powerful tool for gathering thoughts, opinions, feelings and attitudes on particular issues. Focus groups give rich data as they not only give data from individuals in a group, but they also provide data that result from the group dynamics or the interactions in the group. Ideas put forward by one member of the group may serve to spark a train of thought or response for another group member and a good facilitator may be able to work with the group through a process of building on ideas and concepts. Focus groups, therefore, have the advantage of using group dynamics to stimulate discussion, gain insights and generate ideas in order to pursue a topic in greater depth (Bowling, 2000). They can be used to examine not only what people think, but how they think and why they think in that way, their understandings and priorities (Kitzinger, 1995). Focus groups are useful for exploring values about health and disease (see Mc Auliffe, 1996; Mc Auliffe and Ntata, 1994) and are used extensively in market research and health promotion and action research. The group processes can help people to explore their views and generate questions in ways that they would find more difficult in face-to-face interviews (Kitzinger, 1996).

It is important to distinguish between focus groups and action groups. The purpose of focus groups is to gather exploratory data; the purpose of action groups is to plan and take action. However, it is important to be aware that focus groups may unintentionally result in action. For example, a focus group with cancer patients may result in some of the participants realising the value of sharing experiences and deciding to establish a support group.

Critical Incidents in OD

Critical incidents are incidents or events that are critical to the person's view of a particular phenomenon or problem. Flanagan (1954: 341) first described the critical incidents technique as a "flexible set of procedures for collecting direct observations of human behaviour in such a way as to facilitate their potential usefulness in solving practical problems and developing broad psychological principles". It is a technique that is commonly used for collecting incidents that the respondent feels have been critical to his/her experience of a job. Once the incident has been recorded the interviewer then uses probing questions to elicit the details of the incident and the respondent's reactions and feelings about the incident. Further exploration can reveal the skills that are important to the respondent's performance in such situations. Used in this way the technique can be a powerful tool for identifying individual development needs, i.e. how the respondent needs to develop in order to do his/her job more effectively. MacLachlan and Mc Auliffe (1993) make use of the technique to elicit the job-related abilities and characteristics necessary for counselling refugees. It has particular merit in OD interventions as it facilitates the participation of employees in identifying development needs and required job characteristics. It can also be useful in identifying competencies and designing training programmes.

Observation in OD

For OD practitioners and managers, the primary data generation comes through active involvement in the day-to-day organisational processes relating to the change project. Not only are data generated through participation in and observation of teams at work, problems being solved, decisions being made and so on, but also through the interventions that are made to advance the project. Some of these observations and interventions are made in formal settings, such as meetings and interviews; many are made in informal settings, such as over coffee, lunch and other recreational settings.

When OD practitioners observe the dynamics of groups at work – for example, communication patterns, leadership behaviour, use of power, group roles, norms, elements of culture, problem solving and decision making, relations with other groups – they are provided with the basis for inquiry into the underlying assumptions and their effects on the work and life of these groups (Schein, 1999b). As they are dealing with directly observable phenomena in the organisations with which they are working, the critical issue for them is how to inquire into what they are observing and, at the same time, be helpful to the system. For example, at a team meeting they may notice all sorts of behaviour that they suspect might affect how the team goes about its work – people not listening to each other, wandering off the agenda and so on. If they make an intervention into these areas they are aiming to focus on what is useful for the advancement of the change project, rather than what they have observed.

Without this discipline they may reflect what they have observed, but the observation may not be owned by participants in the system because it does not meet their needs or it appears to be showing how clever the OD practitioner is in observing these things. For example, the OD practitioner is observing a resource allocation meeting of the community care team, the purpose of which is to devise a more equitable resource allocation system or method. The discussion and dynamics of the group suggest to the OD practitioner that two of the members of the group used the existing system to their advantage and the other members of the group are angry because the two departments concerned have consistently been allocated most resources. The OD practitioner may suggest this to the group and find that the group unanimously denies that this is the case. It may be that the group is well aware of this problem, but realises that raising it now will serve only to alienate the two departments concerned and make it more difficult for the group to agree a new system.

Rapid Appraisal in OD

Action researchers and development workers often use rapid appraisal techniques to gain a quick assessment of the local community's views and perceptions and the problems they wish to address. The technique is based on interviews with key people and group meetings (Ong, 1993). The aim of rapid appraisal is to gain insight quickly into the population of interest and to gain insight into the community's own perspectives of its needs (Bowling, 2000). Its advantage is its greater speed in comparison with other methods. The method is validated through triangulation. In the initial phases multi-stakeholder meetings are held to determine the topics for study and the appropriate research methods. The research phase may include demographic profiling, household surveys, focus groups and so on. The final phase involves multi-stakeholders in summarising the findings and deciding on actions. It is a useful approach for OD as it facilitates participation in diagnosing problems and planning action. It can be particularly useful in situations that require rapid action or in large-scale change where it may not be possible to involve a large group of organisational members throughout the complete OD intervention. For example, if a series of medication errors had occurred in a short time-span in a particular clinical setting, rapid appraisal provides a means of exploring the issues, diagnosing the problems and initiating a solution within a relatively short space of time – something which is clearly crucial when lives are at stake.

Delphi Technique in OD

The technique involves the use of a group of people who have expertise in the subject under study to generate and refine concepts that help to deepen understanding of the issue (Bowling, 2000). The methods usually, but not always, involve a postal questionnaire method that uses open-ended questions to obtain the ideas, attitudes or opinions of a number of people anonymously. The ideas from the first stage are analysed and fed back to the same people for further comment or refinement. The feedback may be used to develop a set of statements on the topic and these are then fed back to the experts again, asking them to rank their level of agreement with each statement. The process continues until consensus is reached on most of the items. This method has been used to establish health priorities.

The Delphi technique can also be used with a face-to-face group. For example an OD consultant may want to identify the nature and details of a particular problem. He might take the following steps:

1. Bring together a group of people who are affected by the problem and briefly describe the problem as he understands it.
2. Ask each member of the group to independently write down three factors that they believe are contributing to the problem (they should be able to justify these).
3. Collect these factors and distribute them to the whole group.
4. Ask the group to comment on others' lists and revise their own in light of what they have received.
5. Repeat the process until a consensus is reached in the group as to the main factors contributing to the problem.

Nominal Group Technique in OD

This process involves a group of people coming together having been asked to decide their views on a topic in advance of meeting (Bowling, 2000). Their views are fed back to the group and each member is asked to rank the ideas. The results are summarised and fed back in a subsequent meeting. At this meeting they discuss the rankings and their differences. Following this discussion they are asked to re-rank the issues in light of the group's discussion. The final analyses of the re-rankings are fed back to the participants. This method could be used by an OD facilitator in a situation where several courses of action have been proposed in the implementation of a change project. The nominal group technique could help to identify the best course of action for the team or it could be used to prioritise a set of actions.

USING DATA TO DIAGNOSE ORGANISATIONS

Underlying the principle of organisational diagnosis is a notion of organisational health, which organisational clinicians are using to compare with the present situation or ill health (Schein, 1997). Accordingly, frameworks that postulate key organisational variables and relationships are important diagnostic tools (Harrison, 1994; Howard, 1994; Harrison and Shirom, 1999). Organisational frameworks are presentations of organisations which help categorise data, enhance understanding, interpret data and provide a common shorthand language and help guide action for change (Burke, 2002). They typically describe relationships between organisational dynamics, such as purpose, strategy, structure, control systems, information systems, rewards systems and culture, and help organise data into useful categories and point to what areas need attention. We presented the Burke-Litwin and organisational levels models in chapters 4 and 5 as useful and relevant diagnostic frameworks.

Some guidelines are useful for selecting and using frameworks. Weisbord (1988) advises that frameworks should have four features: that they be simple, fit members' values and highlight things they consider important, validate members' experience by putting recognisable things in a new light and that they suggest practical steps. Burke (2002) provides three guidelines for selecting a framework. The first is that you should adopt a framework you understand and with which you feel comfortable. The second is that the framework selected should fit the organisation as closely as possible, that it be comprehensive enough to cover as many aspects of the organisation as appropriate and that it be clear enough for members of the organisation to grasp. The third is that the framework should be sufficiently comprehensive to enable data gathering and interpretation without omitting key pieces of information. In a word of caution, Burke points out two caveats. The first is that a model is only as good as the components selected and the arrangement of these components, and the second is that one may become trapped by one's frameworks, so that one's way of seeing becomes a way of not seeing. OD practitioners need to critique the frameworks they use.

DATA GENERATION AS INTERVENTION

In action research and OD, data can be generated through intervention. Therefore, it is important to know that acts intended to collect data are themselves interventions. So asking an individual a question or observing him/her at work is not simply collecting data but is also *generating* learning data for both the OD practitioner and the individual concerned. Every action, even the very intention and the presence involved in collecting data, is an intervention and has political implications across the system. Accordingly, it is more appropriate to speak of data *generation* than data gathering or collection.

In considering the use of a survey instrument, OD practitioners keep an eye on the organisational dynamics that accompany a survey. While surveying employees by questionnaire as to their views on some aspects of their work or the organisation tends to be seen merely as a method of collecting information, it is more important to see how it is an intervention. A junior doctor's reaction to being asked to participate in an interview may be as informative about the hospital's culture as the responses themselves. Mc Auliffe and MacLachlan (1992) highlight clinicians' resistance to a consumer satisfaction survey in mental health services. In a subsequent paper they advocate the importance of including all clinicians in the design phase of such research and point out that asking for suggestions may not be sufficient, as "those who offer no suggestions are just as able to sabotage the research as those clinicians who have made an active contribution" (MacLachlan and Mc Auliffe, 1992: 52). The reception of a questionnaire by employees may generate questioning, suspicion, anxiety, enthusiasm – all of which are real data for OD practitioners and managers as to what is really going on. If they ignore this they may be missing a key element of how the organisational problem exists and does not get solved, and indeed what issues lie ahead in the change process.

In a similar vein, interviewing in action research and OD is not simply a tool for collecting data. As we have pointed out, asking someone a question or a series of questions is a data-generating intervention. The effect of the question "Why do you choose to work here?" on a ward sister in a hospital may be sufficient to cause her to reflect on her own values and behaviour, and resolve to change them, perhaps by attempting to gain more satisfaction from her job or by leaving to work in a more enriching environment.

DATA-BASED FEEDBACK

Data-based feedback is based on assumptions that information energises and directs behaviour (Nadler, 1977). Data-based information is information that is gathered in a systematic way and analysed professionally. It can be contrasted with hearsay, where people generalise on what "everybody thinks" without any validation. Information arouses energy and affects perception, both positively and negatively. Information can be false and can mislead, misdirect energy and lead to defensive behaviour. Accordingly, while feeding back data to members of an organisation is intended to motivate and direct, it may have the opposite effect. Therefore, an important element of OD work is how diagnosis is acted on and how data are collected and fed back to members of an organisation.

Survey Feedback Method

As early as 1947, questionnaire surveys were being used to assess employee morale and attitudes. A study initiated by Likert and conducted by Floyd Mann at this time used survey data to improve performance at the Edison Company in Detroit, USA. Mann (1957, cited in Burke, 2002) through this work developed a method of improving organisational performance that is now known as "survey feedback". Mann noticed that when a manager was given the survey results, improvement depended on what he did with these results. If the manager shared the results with subordinates, positive changes usually ensued. If he did not share the results, typically nothing happened. Mann believed that survey results should be fed back systematically, starting at the top and flowing downward through the organisational hierarchy in what he termed the "interlocking chain of conferences". Each functional unit or department within the organisation should receive general feedback pertaining to the whole organisation and specific feedback on its own group. Following a discussion of the meaning of the results for the group, they then jointly plan action steps for improvement.

Likert in 1967 built on this process to develop his "Profile of Organisational Characteristics", a questionnaire and model containing six sections: leadership, motivation, communication, decisions, goals and control (Likert, 1967). These were surveyed within a framework of four organisational systems: System 1 – Autocratic; System 2 – Benevolent Autocracy; System 3 – Consultative; and System 4 – Participative and Consensus Management. Likert argued that System 4 was the most desirable and that most employees would agree. Likert was therefore able to develop a profile of an organisation according to the four types along his six organisational dimensions. Survey feedback is beneficial and powerful, according to Burke (2002), for the following reasons:

- It is based on data.
- It involves an organisation's members directly.
- It provides information on what to change and in which priority.
- It focuses change towards the larger system, not at individuals *per se*.

Nadler (1977) presents a cycle for using data-based methods. This cycle comprises five steps:

1. Planning to collect data.
2. Systematically collecting data.
3. Analysing data.

4. Feeding back data.
5. Following up.

Planning to Collect Data

For the OD practitioner there are a number of key issues. First, there are issues around relationship building and contracting which involve working with the client on the goals of the OD project, the approaches to be used, clarifying expectations and building understanding and commitment. Second, there are issues around deciding what kinds of data to collect and how to collect them. Third, there are issues around developing plans for feeding back the data and for how to use the data building commitment to follow through. Fourth, there are issues around evaluation and how the OD project will be evaluated.

Collecting Data

Data are collected for three goals: to obtain valid information, to create and direct energy, and to build relationships. In order to collect data from potential respondents OD practitioners need to clarify a number of issues. These typically include who they are, why they are here and doing what they are doing, whom they work for, what they want from the respondents and why, how they will protect the confidentiality of the respondents, who will have access to the data, what the respondents will get from participating and whether they can be trusted.

There are three basic data-collection techniques – interviews, questionnaires and observation. Each of these techniques has a set of issues and skills. In interviewing, choosing between structured, semi-structured or unstructured approaches, learning how to conduct an interview and how to code responses are some of the critical skills to be learned. In using questionnaires, one can choose between using an already existing instrument and designing one's own. With regard to the latter, questionnaire design is a sophisticated field. Trust issues are particularly pertinent to observation approaches, whether formal or unobtrusive.

Each technique has its own advantages and disadvantages. For instance, interviewing is very time consuming and can be expensive; questionnaires are impersonal and confine respondents to answering the questions they are asked. Choosing what technique to use requires considerable thought.

An important frame of mind for OD practitioners is that there is no such thing as mere data collection. All data gathering is an intervention and of itself generates data. A questionnaire may generate:

*   *Apathy*: "Here comes another survey. Nothing comes from these."
*   *Suspicion or hostility*: "A lot of people lost their job after the last survey."

- *Anxiety*: "What are they really after? Be careful about what we answer."
- *Anticipation/hope*: "At last they are asking for our views. Maybe now something will happen."

For OD practitioners such reactions are real and relevant data, and provide valuable insight into what is really going on. Sometimes this is the critical data to work on and may mean abandoning or postponing a survey.

Data Analysis

Data analysis is integrally linked to the planning phase. Unless one has decided in advance why one is collecting the data and what it is for, then the analysis will be a confusing and confused activity. There are two components of data analysis. First, there is a conceptual frame that provides some model of organisational functioning, such as discussed in the earlier part of this chapter. This provides some sort of map for analysing the data. Second, there are the technical tools, which enable OD practitioners to have confidence that the answers received are reliable patterns of answer to the questions asked.

Data Feedback

Feeding data back to a client group is an important process concern for OD practitioners. They know that information can be de-energising or divisive; they know that the process of how data is communicated is critical to whether the data is actually understood and accepted or not. There are many ways of presenting data: in a quantitative format, in a written report and in feedback meetings. While the written formats are likely to be required for formal purposes, OD practitioners are likely to prefer feedback meetings because they provide further data of what is going on in the organisation and provide an opportunity for continuing intervention.

There are two criteria in determining the order in which data are fed back (Neilsen, 1984). The first is rank. OD practitioners' contract is likely to stipulate that those more powerful need to see the data first. That allows senior managers to prepare for their subordinates' responses and also to check (and perhaps veto) how the data is to be fed back to the rest of the organisation. Accordingly, OD practitioners need to build commitment to the data feedback process by involving the more powerful all through the process. The second criterion is the general relevance of the data to particular sections of the organisation. The groups to which the data are presented must be appropriate to the issues and must have appropriate power to deal with the issues arising from the data. So a case may be made that different groups may be exposed to different parts of the data.

The attendants at the meeting may feel anxiety, defensiveness, fear or hope about the presentation of the data. They may question the validity of the data, they may resist accepting responsibility for the data and what they represent. Individuals may express:

- *Denial and even outrage*: "We don't really have any problems." "It is dangerous to print this."
- *Attack on the respondents*: "Of course they said that. They never..."
- *Scepticism*: "Just watch. Nothing will happen."
- *Apathy*: "We knew this already".
- *Platitudes*: "It's good to have all this in the open." "We need this."
- *Interest*: "Why would some say...?" "What does this mean?"

Nadler (1977) suggest some important meeting processes:

- Help people be motivated to work with the data.
- Assist them to use the data.
- Have a structure for the meeting.

Following Up

This is the crucial stage for the OD practitioner because in OD and action research data are not collected, analysed and fed back solely for the pursuit of new knowledge or because they are interesting in themselves. They are collected, analysed and fed back in order to enable change take place. This change does not just happen of its own accord. It needs to be planned and implemented. Decisions need to be taken on whether to initiate a new intervention, cease, continue, or expand an existing intervention. Examples of following-up activities would be action planning or in some instances identifying the need to collect more data.

DATA AND EVALUATION

What is Evaluation?

Evaluation is "a set of planned, information-gathering and analytical activities undertaken to provide those responsible for the management of change with a satisfactory assessment of the effects and/or progress of the change effort" (Beckhard and Harris, 1977: 86). This definition broadens the activities beyond data collection to analytical activities and also identifies the need to assess/evaluate the *process* of change as well as the outcomes or impact. It is important to view evaluation as an OD-inquiry process that contributes to organisational change and learning and not solely as a mechanical tool for assessing outcomes (Preskill and Torres, 1999). Just as data gathering is an intervention so too is evaluation.

Why Evaluate?

There are many reasons that may be put forward for not evaluating OD work, amongst them, "It's too difficult and complex", "You can't control all the variables in an organisation", "It's difficult to measure shifts in attitude", "Most of the changes are process changes and not easily observable" and so on. Despite these difficulties there are several compelling reasons why one should evaluate OD interventions:

1. Evaluation pushes OD practitioners to clearly define the objectives or goals of the intervention.
2. Evaluation dictates that OD practitioners have clear outcomes defined for the intervention.
3. Evaluation necessitates a shared understanding of how the outcomes are to be measured.
4. Evaluation calls for the documentation of how certain procedures, events and activities will be implemented.
5. Evaluation helps to identify many of the problems or barriers that might arise in the implementation of the OD intervention.
6. Evaluation facilitates planning for the next steps or intervention in the on-going effort to improve organisational effectiveness.

What to Evaluate

Evaluating Organisational Learning

Organisational learning refers to how organisations as systems learn, rather than how its individuals learn. Individual learning does not necessarily transfer to organisational learning (Coghlan, 1997). Senge's (1990) distinction between "generative" and "adaptive" learning is a distinction between the capacity for an organisation to reinvent itself, re-examine and evolve its assumptions, and to test them against new realities (generative learning), not merely to improve its capacity to adapt efficiently (adaptive learning). As learning is a social process that occurs best in a group setting where the group is engaged in pursuit of a common and relevant task, the ability to engage in dialogue is central to organisational learning.

Organisational learning is intrinsic to OD and one of the key aims of OD interventions is to stimulate organisational learning. Therefore, any evaluation of OD should "measure" organisational learning. What has the organisation learnt as a result of the OD intervention? Has the OD intervention improved the organisation's learning capacity and learning ability? These are some of the questions that OD evaluations should be attempting to answer.

Evaluating Understanding
In some evaluations, the main reason for commissioning an evaluation study may be to increase the audience's conceptual understanding of the influence of a social intervention in which it has an interest. Thus enlightenment is the end-point in the evaluation–utilisation chain (Owen and Lambert, 1995)

Evaluating for Programme Modification
Owen (1993) describes an approach to evaluation, which he calls "evaluation in programme management". This approach stems from the work of Joseph Wholey who derived a set of approaches to evaluation. He worked interactively with managers to fine-tune programmes. As evaluator he provided information by which the implementation and the outcomes of that programme could be monitored over time. A key feature of this approach was the provision of timely information for decisions about programme modification. Evaluators should be prepared to contribute evaluation information at any stage of the development of a given programme (Stufflebeam, 2000). Preskill and Torres (1999) highlight that in addition to this, evaluators have a role to play in assembling evaluative information throughout the programme to celebrate organisational successes and reinforce learning.

Evaluating to Influence Leaders
Owen and Lambert (1995) suggest that evaluators are in a unique position to influence the mental models of leaders and influence decision making and organisational learning. They have the opportunity through systematic data collection and feedback to gain insight into programme and system dynamics. An evaluator who adopts this position:

- Consciously builds into evaluation design opportunities to move across system boundaries.
- Actively encourages design and clarification of evaluation at the planning, trial and early implementation phases, before the programme becomes too entrenched and resistant to change.
- Develops methods of data collection and reporting that will contribute directly to informing and challenging leaders' understanding of the organisation and the structure as well as the assumptions and values of the OD programme. (1995: 248)

Evaluating Different Perspectives
An implicit assumption of much OD evaluation is that it is possible to obtain average ratings of the effectiveness of an intervention on predetermined criteria. However, Ramirez and Bartunek (1989) argue that ratings assessed on criteria established before the programme

commences may miss many of the experiences and outcomes of the intervention, such as organisational change unrelated to the original criteria, increased conflict among groups, increased political behaviour and so on. A second problem they identify is the inappropriateness of average ratings in a setting with multiple realities. "They cancel out rather than register differences of opinion among subgroups...it is essential to report results of interventions in such a way that the variety of different reactions can be included" (1989: 54). They conclude that in situations where there are multiple realities, "regardless of the extent to which the intervention acknowledges and addresses these multiple realities, and is successful by some criteria, there is unlikely to be a totally shared perception of its value" (1989: 54).

Evaluating Organisational Effectiveness

The purpose of OD interventions tends to be to improve organisations or make them more effective. Therefore, in order to evaluate OD interventions we need to be clear about what we mean by organisational effectiveness. Cameron (1980) points out that there are at least four criteria for organisational effectiveness and that they differ significantly from one organisation to another.

1. The goal model defines organisational effectiveness in terms of the extent to which the organisation accomplishes its goals.
2. The system resource model defines organisational effectiveness as the ability to acquire much needed resources.
3. The process model defines organisational effectiveness in terms of how smoothly the organisation functions. The Burke-Litwin and interlevels frameworks presented in chapters 4 and 5 provide indicators as to how transformational and transactional factors relate to each other while the interlevels framework points to how the tasks at the individual, team, interdepartmental group and organisation levels need to be in harmony.
4. The strategic constituencies model defines organisational effectiveness as the extent to which the organisation satisfies all its strategies constituencies – special interest groups or stakeholders.

How to Evaluate

Rothwell, Sullivan and McLean (1995) recommend a cyclical approach to evaluation, with the evaluation forming an integral part of the intervention. They suggest the use of formative, summative or longitudinal evaluations. *Formative evaluation* is conducted during the intervention and helps to guide the process; *summative evaluation* is conducted at the end of an intervention, i.e. immediately after completion; and *longitudinal evaluation* is conducted at a specified time after the intervention has been completed. A formative evaluation can be particularly useful in assessing progress and helping to plan or re-plan future phases of the intervention. Summative evaluation may be useful in assessing the impact of the evaluation on the participants, but is also useful in examining process variables (as the process is likely to be fresh in participants' minds immediately after the intervention is completed). Longitudinal evaluations are necessary to assess outcome variables.

Rothwell et al. (1995) also distinguish between OD evaluations in terms of the target. The target of evaluation may be the total organisation or system, the organisation's relationship with other organisations or the outside world, inter-team and intra-team development, interpersonal development, individual development and role development. These targets correspond to the organisational levels we described in chapter 5.

In planning any evaluation, it is important that it is factored in at the design stage of the intervention. The evaluation should be discussed with the client or key stakeholders at the design stage, so that consensus can be reached as to the purpose of the evaluation, at what level it should be targeted and what is to be measured. We have already highlighted some of the issues pertaining to the evaluation's purpose.

It is also important at the design stage to consider what depth of evaluation might be most appropriate. OD practitioners may simply want to gauge reaction to the intervention, i.e. how satisfied are the participants, the clients and so on. They may want to examine what learning has taken place as a result of the intervention (particularly if it is a training intervention) or they may want to delve deeper than attitude and evaluate at the level of behavioural change, i.e. has the intervention resulted in a change in how people actually work. Their clients or the managers in the organisation will probably be most interested in evaluation of the organisational impact of this change, i.e. the improvements in organisational effectiveness resulting from the intervention.

Ideally OD practitioners would evaluate at each level or depth. However, time or budget rarely allows this luxury. It is important that they push to evaluate at the deepest level that time and money will allow. Studies consistently show that management most prefers information on organisational impact and least prefers reaction evaluation only. Therefore, if they want to impress on management the value of OD interventions they should be striving for organisational impact evaluations coupled with evaluation that increases understanding of the process or intervention programme.

Ownership
Involvement of the client and key stakeholders in designing the evaluation is crucial if OD practitioners want cooperation in obtaining accurate data. An understanding of what they are measuring as well as why and how

they are measuring it and what the data will be used for needs to be communicated to all involved. The establishment of a feedback mechanism to enable them to discuss the data throughout the intervention and evaluation is also important. The presentation of the final evaluation should not be an occasion to spring surprises on the client(s). Instead the client(s) should be kept fully informed and involved throughout the evaluation process.

The evaluation should, therefore, be an integral part of the intervention, not something that is separate. Taking an action research approach to OD interventions will ensure that this occurs.

CONCLUSIONS

Data collection and feedback are an integral part of OD interventions. Careful planning and sensitivity are the key skills required to make effective use of data in OD interventions. We have shown how data can be used for several purposes, from planning and preparing for change, assessing progress, influencing programmatic changes, impacting on attitudes or behaviour, providing learning opportunities, influencing leader decision making and planning, to demonstrating organisational learning and the outcomes and impact of interventions.

The multiple realities of organisational life need to be factored into the evaluation of any OD interventions. This is achieved by obtaining data from multiple perspectives using a variety of methods that allow cross-checking and enable the evaluator to build an integrated picture that tells the story of these multiple realities in a manner that is meaningful and useful to the organisation in facilitating its understanding and progress.

Data collection is not a once off event at the end of a programme. Instead it is a continuous process and may form part of a formative, summative or longitudinal evaluation. Evaluation should aim to stimulate organisational learning and to measure the learning capacity within the organisation. Process variables and qualitative data are as important as outcome variables and quantitative data in building a picture that increases organisational understanding of the change process.

Case 6.1 The Medical Cards Issue

The community care service in the Northern Health Board has recently received several complaints from patients, patients' relatives and political representatives complaining on behalf of patients, all of which pertain to inequities in the system of medical card allocation. Medical

cont/d

cards are allocated based on the recipient's income with those below a certain income being automatically entitled to a medical card. The Health Board uses its discretion to occasionally allocate medical cards to those above the threshold on the grounds that they can be classified as "hardship cases". The Northern Health Board's community care services are divided into three geographical areas and each of these areas operates independently when it comes to day-to-day operations and tasks such as allocating medical cards. The recent complaints suggest that there may be differences in the criteria applied to the "hardship cases" in each of the geographical areas. The programme manager with overall responsibility for the service is known to be in favour of centralising the service and increasing the use of IT in decision making, i.e. establishing a range of criteria to complement the income level criterion, and through the use of such criteria identifying eligibility for medical cards. The geographical managers are not entirely in favour of this suggestion as they suspect it would have implications for the centralisation of other services and probably eventually impact on their own positions. The staff are very reluctant to support such a plan, as they state that the service will become depersonalised and the patients will suffer. However, there is also the issue of the geographical movement of staff that might be necessary with a more centralised approach.

Questions
1. Design an OD intervention that uses data to diagnose the problem and provide ongoing feedback to staff in a manner that will facilitate whatever changes may be necessary to address the problems in the service.
2. How would you build an evaluation component into the intervention?

Clinical Inquiry Exercise 6.1

1. Thinking about a change process that you are currently involved in, identify how you might use data as intervention to facilitate the process of change.
2. Map out who the intervention is aimed at and what reaction the data is likely to evoke.
3. Develop a plan for working with the reactions you anticipate.

CHAPTER 7

Large System Change and Learning

"Large system" typically refers to a system of a size beyond that of an individual or small group. In this chapter we apply the principles of OD to how a large system can go about planned change.

> A large system change strategy is a plan defining *what* interventions to make *where*, by *whom* and at what *time* in order to move the system to a state where it can optimally transform need into results in a social environment that nutures peoples' worth and dignity.
> (Beckhard and Harris, 1977: 15)

Why Do Organisations Change?

In systems theory, living systems go through the process of entropy, which essentially means that they go through stages of birth, growth, maturity, decline and death. Organisations as living systems need to thwart the entropic process in order to continue to exist and flourish. Hence, we can speak of negative entropy as meaning an organisation's drive to halt the process of entropy and renew itself (Katz and Kahn, 1978). In more specific terms, technological innovations, government policy and changing customer needs and demands create an imperative for change in contemporary organisations. For health organisations, advances in medical technology, development of new drug therapies, demands for greater accountability at regional and local level and increasing public expectations create the imperative for change.

Why Do Change Efforts Fail?

There have been many critiques of the failures of change programmes to deliver. Beer, Eisenstat and Spector (1990) state bluntly that from their research the reason why most change programmes do not work is because the programmes are guided by a flawed theory of change. In their view, this flawed theory is based on the belief that change needs to begin with changing individuals' knowledge and attitudes which then leads to changes in behaviour which will in turn lead to organisational change. They explain that as individual behaviour is powerfully shaped by the organisational roles that people play, the most effective way to change behaviour is to put people into a new organisational context, which imposes new roles, responsibilities and relationships on them.

Kotter (1995) in contrast, identifies eight errors: not establishing a great enough sense of urgency; not creating a powerful enough guiding coalition; lacking a vision; under-communicating the vision by a factor of ten; not removing obstacles to the new vision; not systematically planning for and creating short-term wins; declaring victory too soon; and not anchoring change in the organisation's culture.

Hamblin, Keep and Ash (2001) focus on management failings: not knowing the fundamental principles of change management; succumbing to the temptations of the "quick fix" and "simple solutions"; not fully appreciating the significance of leadership and cultural aspects of change; not appreciating sufficiently the significance of the people issues; not knowing the critical contribution that the human resource development function can make to the management of change and how trainers and developers lack credibility in the eyes of line managers.

The failures of specific change approaches, such as business process reengineering (BPR), the total quality management (TQM) and IT-driven change to deliver are well-documented (Buchanan, 1997). In the health system, much effort has been focused on management development with the aim of improving services. Yet "the widespread acceptance of traditional custom and practice, and an unwillingness to challenge how things are done are real impediments to change" (Dixon and Baker, 1996: 5). Clearly then, changing the knowledge and attitudes of managers is not enough. The environment in which those managers work must allow them to practice and develop their newly learned skills and behaviours.

> The integration of personal and organisational objectives is a notoriously difficult task but a systematic approach to training and development provides a powerful source of integration. (Dixon and Baker, 1996: 5)

LARGE SYSTEM CHANGE IN HEALTHCARE

In a review of the literature on large-scale organisational and managerial change in healthcare in recent times, Ferlie (1997: 186) identified the commonalities. These included:

- A broad vision rather than a detailed blueprint at the beginning of the process.
- The provision of a visible focus of central and local leadership to drive key changes.
- The creation of new forms of organisation and intermediate tiers in

"green field sites" uncontaminated by the old culture, and setting clear targets for these new tiers.
* Identifying and intervening in "receptive sites" before implementing the intervention in less receptive sites.
* Establishment of early successes, which helped signal that there was no going back.

Pettigrew, Ferlie and McKee (1992) conducted a longitudinal research study on eight Regional Health Authorities in the NHS over a four-year period. They were particularly interested in why the rate and pace of change differs across different localities. They believe that some contexts or environments are more receptive to change than others. They revealed eight receptivity factors as being important determinants of the success of the change process:

1. *Quality and coherence of policy.* The quality of policy generated at local level was found to be important, both from an analytical as well as a process perspective. Using data to substantiate the case for change, and framing this data within clear conceptual thinking, was equally important. Strong testing of initial thoughts was important in ensuring that there was coherence between the proposed strategic framework and the goals of the organisation.

2. *Availability of key people leading change.* Strong leadership from the key change agents coupled with continuity were considered important. They draw evidence from the literature of the link between the unplanned movement of key personnel and the draining of energy, purpose, commitment and action from major change processes. They suggest that a corollary of this problem is "that the change process or programme then goes into a period of regression leaving the newcomer manager to start again but now possibly in a soured and non-receptive context for change" (1992: 278).

3. *Long-term environmental pressure.* They argue that contrary to the idea that large-scale environmental pressure can act as a trigger for or driver of change, in the NHS excessive pressure can deflect or drain energy out of the system. In some of the districts studied, financial crises created delay, denial, collapse of morale, and scapegoating and defeat of managers. In others, financial crisis was played up and skilfully orchestrated by management in order to accelerate the process of rationalisation and change.

4. *A supportive organisational culture.* Culture change is an aspect of change that requires huge energy. Pettigrew et al. (1992) argue that "rewards, broadly defined may be important, and that there is an extremely important role for Human Resource Management policies

and practices, somewhat neglected perhaps in the NHS in the past" (1992: 281). Health services organisations are not characterised by a single culture, but a whole myriad of subcultures. Pettigrew et al. identified a number of features of the managerial subculture at district level that were associated with a high rate of change:

- Flexible working across boundaries with purpose-designed structures rather than traditional hierarchies.
- Openness to research and evaluation.
- A strong value base that helps to give focus to what otherwise might be a loose network.
- Strong positive self-image and a sense of achievement.

5. *Effective managerial-clinical relationships.* The importance of effective managerial-clinical relations in stimulating strategic change has been reported in studies of the US healthcare system. Manager-clinician relations in the NHS study were found to be easier where negative stereotypes had been broken down. This can happen with the emergence of mixed roles, i.e. clinicians with a managerial role. It is important that managers understand what clinicians value, as this will allow them to negotiate or trade more successfully with them. Pettigrew et al. identify clinical directors as strategic clinicians that are critical people for management to identify, foster and encourage, and that "under no circumstances should they be driven into opposition by trivia" (1992: 283).

6. *Cooperative inter-organisational networks.* The most effective networks with other agencies were those that were both informal and purposeful. The significance of purposeful networks and their role in trust building, and negotiating is something important to achieving substantive change.

7. *Simplicity and clarity of goals and priorities.* It is important to be able to narrow the change agenda down to a key set of priorities and to be patient in pursuing these over a long period of time. If the constantly shifting short-term pressures in the NHS cause an escalation in the number of priorities there is a danger that they may become meaningless to the organisation.

8. *The fit between the district's change agenda and its locale.* There are a number of factors that proved important to the Districts' plans for change including: whether there was one large population centre or two or more; whether there was a teaching hospital presence; the nature of the local NHS workforce; and the strength and nature of the local political culture.

Enacting Large System Change

Richard Beckhard has long been considered one of the founders of organisation development and the creator of the core framework for large system change (Beckhard, 1969, 1997b). He articulated a generic change framework, which in its essence comprises four main themes:

1. Determining the need for change.
2. Articulating a desired future.
3. Assessing the present and what needs to be changed in order to move to the desired future.
4. Getting to the desired future by managing the transition. (Beckhard and Harris, 1987; Beckhard and Pritchard, 1992)

An additional feature is the role external help might play in the process, a subject we will deal with in chapter 10. Beckhard's framework has been acknowledged as the core model from which other models have been adapted (e.g. Nadler, 1998; Cummings and Worley, 2001).

In Beckhard's view, any change process involves a current state with which there is dissatisfaction and initial unfreezing, and hence a perceived need for change. There is a *desired future state*, which is the desired and planned outcome of the change process. There is also the *transition state*, which is the interim period of time and state of affairs that exists between identifying the need for change and achieving it.

We are extending Beckhard's framework and drawing on Nadler's (1998) development of it by naming a five-phase change process cycle:

1. Determining the need for change.
2. Defining the desired future state.
3. Assessing the present in terms of the desired future to determine the changes to be made.
4. Implementing the change and managing the transition.
5. Consolidating and sustaining the change.

Determining the Need for Change

The preferred starting place is to inquire into the context for change in the organisation, unit or subunit (Pettigrew, 1987). The change process begins with an acknowledgement of the need for change, or as Nadler puts it "recognising the change imperative" (1998: 75). It may seem obvious that naming the need for change and its causes is essential. The forces for change may be coming from the external environment, such as government policy. In healthcare, external forces include demands for greater accountability and value for money, political demands for locally accessible healthcare, increased consumer knowledge as a result of the

Figure 7.1 The Process of Large System Change

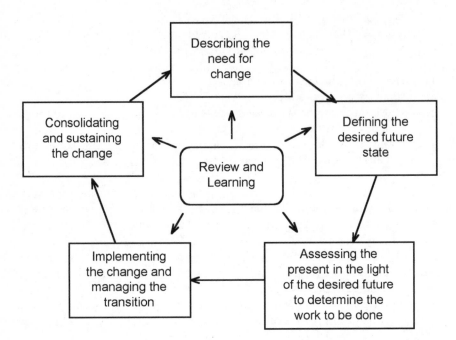

vast amounts of healthcare information available on the internet, labour market and recruitment problems. They may come from internal forces, such as budget over-runs, low morale among staff, excessive dysfunctional political inter-group rivalry, the needs of a diverse work force, increasing demands for accountability, quality, the need for managers to move from "command and control" styles of management typically associated with bureaucratic and hierarchical forms of organisation to styles that value building collaborative relations within teams and working laterally rather than vertically across organisations. In healthcare current internal forces for change include high staff turnover, staff shortages and technological advances influencing the practice of consultants and so on. The analysis of these forces identifies their source, their potency and the nature of the demands they are making on the system. These forces for change need to be assessed so that major ones are distinguished from minor ones, symptoms from causes and so on.

A second key element in evaluating the need for change is the degree of choice about whether to change or not. This is often an overlooked question. Choices are not absolute. While there may be no control over the forces demanding change, there is likely to be a great deal of control over how to respond to those forces. In that case there is likely to be a good deal of scope as to what changes, how and in what time-scale the change can take place.

The outcome of determining the need for change is to ask a further question, which is whether first- or second-order change is required. By first-order change is meant an improvement in what the organisation does or how it does it. By second-order change is meant a system-wide change in the nature of the core assumptions and ways of thinking and acting. The choice of whether to follow a first- or second-order change process may be as much determined by organisational politics as by the issues under consideration. How the key organisational actors interpret the forces for change and how they form their subsequent judgement as to what choices they have are important political dynamics.

There are critical interlevel dynamics in the activities of assessing the need for change (Coghlan, 2000a). The change process has to begin somewhere. Who decides that change is required may be anyone in the organisation. The individual, whether someone in direct dealing with customers or a high-level executive, who first perceives that need for change must have the confidence to take the agenda to those in executive positions and persuade them to adopt his/her insight. If those in the executive positions deny or dodge the relevance of that insight, then the individual may have to present the case for change more forcibly or indeed may retreat. When a management team adopts the need for change and begins to act, it has then to win over other teams in the system. A critical process then is how the imperative for change is communicated across the organisation (Quirke, 1996). Each of these movements – from individual to team to interdepartmental group – is an iterative process (Rashford and Coghlan, 1994). In other words, when the team adopts an individual's position, that adoption reinforces the individual. When other teams adopt a particular team's position, that reinforces that team and, of course, when customers adopt a new service, that reinforces the organisation.

OD practitioners may be utilised at the point where questions are being asked about how to move the need-for-change question through the organisation. Interventions may attend to how individuals and teams perceive the need for change and what their sources of resistance are. Interventions might focus on how internal or external data only are considered, perceptual defences whereby data are distorted, and where different subsystems attend to different data. Critical interventions would focus on building formal structures – planning groups, data-gathering groups, etc. – and inter-functional dialogue where assumptions and perceptions of data are shared and heard.

Defining the Desired Future

Once a sense of the need for change has been established, the most useful focus for attention is to define a desired future state or develop "a shared direction" (Nadler, 1998: 78). This process is essentially that of articulating what the organisation, unit or subunit would look like after change has taken place. This process is critical, as it helps provide focus and energy by describing the desires for the future in a positive light. However, an initial focus on the problematic or imperfect present may over-emphasise negative experiences and generate pessimism. Working at building consensus on a desired future is an important way of harnessing the political elements of the system.

Clearly, the process of defining the future involves interlevel dynamics (Coghlan, 2000a). If the vision comes from the chief executive, then there are interlevel dynamics from that individual to the senior management team and then to the interdepartmental group and on to the organisation. As the CEO takes his vision to the senior team and works at persuading its members to adopt it, the movement is from the individual to the team. If the vision is created by the senior management team then the process begins with the team and moves to individuals within that team, is reinforced in the team and then goes to the interdepartmental group and on to the organisation. So the iteration of issue presentation, reaction and response ebbs and flows from individual to individual, team to team and so on.

Assessing the Present in Terms of the Desired Future to Determine the Necessary Changes

When the desired future state is articulated, the present reality needs to be attended to and the question, "What is it in the present that needs changing in order to move to the desired future state?" needs to be asked. Because the present is being assessed in the light of the desired future, it is assessing what needs changing and what does not. It may judge that for the change to effectively take place, a change in current structures, attitudes, roles, policies or activities may be needed. As any change problem is a cluster of possible changes, it may need to group particular problems under common headings, i.e. HRM policies and practices, service delivery, information management, reward systems, organisational structure and design, and so on. Then it describes the problem more specifically and asks, "Which of these requires priority attention? If A is changed, will a solution to B fall easily into place? What needs to be done first?" This step is about taking a clear, comprehensive, accurate view of the current state of the organisation, involving an organisational diagnosis which names:

- The priorities within the cluster of change problems.
- The relevant subsystems where change is required.
- An assessment of the readiness and capability for the contemplated change.

Another element in describing the present is to describe the relevant parts of the organisation that will be involved in the change. This description points to the critical people needed for the change to take place. This is an explicit consideration of the political system. Examples of who needs to be involved might include specific managers, nursing and medical staff. For example, in designing a new ward or unit, it is important that all professions who will work in or interface with that unit have their views represented to the design team. If the key people are not involved in the design and planning process, there is a danger of discovering the design flaws only after the building is in use and they may prove difficult if not impossible to rectify. The readiness and capability for change of the key people must be assessed. Readiness points to the motivation and willingness to change, while capability refers to whether they are able, psychologically and otherwise, to change.

Interlevel processes are critical to this step (Coghlan, 2000a). Assessment of the present may create defensiveness in individuals, teams and between teams. There may be tendencies to attempt to shift blame for change problems from one team onto another. In assessing readiness and capability, a critical aspect may be how teams are capable or ready, or how much capability and readiness there is between teams. This may refer to political dynamics between teams or to issues such as information management or IT compatibility. "Relevant subsystems" refers to individuals, teams and to the interdepartmental group.

Interventions need to focus on dialogue within teams and between teams to agree on criteria for evaluation of the present strengths and weaknesses, with the accompanying focus on reducing the influence of interdepartmental politics, defensive routines and conflict. A particular focus for such intervention might be dialogue between the different service deliverers. For example, in introducing integrated management units or clinical directorates to a hospital, dialogue needs to take place, not just between nursing, medical and paramedical staff, but also between the different specialties that are likely to be part of the same directorate.

Implementing the Change and Managing the Transition

This step is what is generally perceived as being the actual change process, though as we have seen, preparation for change is equally essential. The critical task is to move from the present to the future and manage the intervening period of transition. The transition state is both a state of affairs and a period of time. As a state of affairs between the present and the future it is typically a difficult time because the past is found to be defective and no longer tenable and the new state has not yet come into being. It is akin to bio-social life-cycle stages like adolescence or retirement. It is an in-between state. For individuals there are feelings of a) instability, because well-established structures, roles, procedures and outcomes are being or have been taken away, b) instability, because what is to replace the former structures, roles and procedures is not yet in position and c) stress, because participants are in an in-between state and trying to manage both the process of changing and the normal activity of service delivery. Consequently, for members of organisations there are issues around anxiety, power and control. Because organisations are political entities, who has power to get others to change and how they use that power, and how that power is experienced by those who carry the brunt of the change are very important issues. As a period of time the transition state marks the time span across weeks, months or years where the change is being implemented through the system. So, in essence, the transition state is a unique state of affairs and duration of time, as the old has gone and the new has not yet been realised, and so needs to be seen and managed as such. It makes pressing psychological demands of members of organisations and also makes demands on those in management and leadership positions. "Business as usual during alterations" is a useful caption for the transition state as it captures the essence of the twin tasks – keeping the service going and changing at the same time.

There are four tasks to managing this transition state. One is having a strategic and operational plan that simply defines the goals, activities, structures, projects and experiments that will help achieve the desired state. A common mistake in large system change is the failure to move from the transition state to the desired state. This may happen because the transition state is mistaken for the end of the intervention. For example, in moving a hospital to a new site, the change process does not end when everyone is in situ. Another reason can be the belief that the desired state, i.e. the consolidation and stabilisation, will take care of itself. For example, a great deal of effort is put into training, but then is never followed up.

The second task is the inclusion of the transition state in the change plan. This means anticipating the critical areas in which transition will be difficult. It involves planning to allocate some resources to the transition plan, perhaps for time devoted to working on transition issues, such as roles, responsibilities, decision making, problem solving, education and training interventions.

The third task of the transition state is its management. If the management of the transition is neglected, as it often is, then the change process may flounder and get bogged down. "Business as usual during alterations" means that the alterations process needs to be managed. There are several ways this can be done. One is that the chief executive or head acts as the change project manager. If this happens then other day-to-day responsibilities need to be delegated so that the manager has the time to give to the change project. Another way to manage the transition is to appoint a change project manager on a temporary assignment. This manager needs to have the clout necessary to mobilise necessary resources, have the respect of key leaders and have good interpersonal skills. A third way is to have a change project group, whether on a hierarchical or representational basis.

The Nursing Education Forum Report (2000) acknowledged the significance of the transition period in the development of the pre-registration nursing degree programme. It suggests that management structures be established at national and local level to implement the report and manage the transition period.

As no amount of change can take place without commitment, the fourth task is a plan to build commitment. The commitment plan focuses on who in the organisation must be committed to the change if it is to take place. There may be particular individuals and groups whose support is a prerequisite for the change and a critical mass whose commitment is necessary to provide the energy and support for the change to occur. Commitment ranges along a scale from a "no commitment" at one extreme to a "make" the change happen at the other. The political dynamics of building commitment of key power groups involves finding areas of agreement and compromise among conflicting views and negotiating cooperation (Fisher and Ury, 1986; Ury, 1991). Those who are leading the change often forget that, while they have had access to information and have been discussing issues for some time, there is a critical mass of members who are not as familiar with the issues or the rationale behind decisions as they are, and who therefore need to be informed and brought into the change process. We know from experience, as well as from social science, that people can deny the need for change and try to dodge it, not because of any malevolence on their part, but because the change issues are new to them and they have not been exposed to them or have not had any opportunity to explore them in depth. We also know that telling people something does not mean that they hear, understand or accept it. Hence, the demands for two-way communication, where change leaders listen as well as inform are critical. As change is being implemented and the transition state is in progress, the need to continuously reinforce the vision of the desired future, listen to the problems that are being thrown up in the transition period and encourage implementation is essential.

Interlevel dynamics are pivotal to the processes of the transition state as individuals and teams address the implications and implementation of the change agenda. As the change agenda affects the work of individuals in what they do and how they do it, individual commitment is essential. As the change agenda affects the work of the permanent teams and typically requires the creation of new teams and work in temporary committees or project groups, team dynamics are critical to the change process. In a similar vein, the change agenda involves the interface of multiple teams with respect to information sharing, problem identification and resolution, resource allocation and collective bargaining, inter-team dynamics can enable or hinder the successful management of the change process.

Building commitment is essentially an interlevel process. Individuals identify with their teams, profession or occupational community or trade union, so efforts to build commitment involve interventions with teams and across teams, particularly if inter-team relations are likely to have a negative impact on the progress of the change.

Consolidating and Sustaining the Change

As is often pointed out, relaxing too soon in the belief that the change has been made is likely to be a very damaging error of judgement. Frequently the hardest work is done in consolidating and sustaining a change, when people might think that the hardest part is over. Consolidation refers to the period immediately after the implementation of the change. There are several key tasks to be done to ensure the change survives and works. The progress of the change needs to be monitored, assessed and refined as necessary in order that the changed state becomes normative and central to the new way of life. The new way of delivering the service needs to be rewarded, small successes, recognised and celebrated. In this phase, the human resource function plays a key role in institutionalising the change. Sustaining the change refers to the longer term and involves aligning the informal organisation with the formal, where people feel good about successful change and experience the dissipation of threat. Of course, this in turn sets up a resistance to further change or diverts attention from making this change work because more change is on the horizon.

REVIEW AND LEARNING

The key to successful change is attention to learning and, as we have seen, the critical dimension to action research is how review is undertaken and managed. Review is essentially reflection on experience and in any such reflection the critical questions are asked, not to evoke guilt or blame, but to generate learning as to what is taking place and what needs to be adjusted. If review is undertaken in this spirit then the likelihood of individual or team defensiveness can be lessened and learning can take place.

LARGE SYSTEM CHANGE AND ORGANISATIONAL LEARNING

In many respects OD and organisational learning are closely related. Argyris' notion of single- and double-loop learning corresponds to first- and second-order change (Argyris and Schon, 1996). The notion of building learning capabilities is well-supported by OD theory and practice (DiBella, 2001).

A distinction between organisational learning and the learning organisation is frequently made. Organisational learning refers to the process of enabling learning to take place in an organisation, while the learning organisation is understood to be the outcome of well-established patterns and habits of organisational learning. OD is seen as an important approach to helping organisations become learning organisations (Watkins and Golembiewski, 2000). The interventions to enable change and learning to happen complement each other. The processes of enacting systemic change in individuals, teams, the interdepartmental group and the organisation are very similar to those of enabling learning (Watkins and Marsick, 1993; Marsick and Watkins, 1999). Organisational learning typically aims to identify the learning that individual members of an organisation have achieved and then to extend that learning to the organisation (Dixon, 1994). But as Coghlan (1997) points out, to go from individual to organisation in one step is a big leap and so he argues for an interlevel approach to enabling individual learning to become team learning and interdepartmental group learning before it can be termed organisational learning.

CONCLUSIONS

In this chapter we have looked at how organisational change efforts fail and emphasised the important role context plays in change. We have explored the notion of enabling a large system to change. We have drawn primarily on the pioneering work of Richard Beckhard whose framework we view as a useful map. It identifies issues, lays out routes and provides valuable headings for change agents, whether managers or OD practitioners, to consider.

Case 7.1 Clinicians in Management Initiative, Part A

The Clinicians in Management Initiative (CIM) was launched in 1998 by the Minister for Health. The aim of this initiative was to give health professionals a greater involvement in planning, management and decision-making within hospitals. It was envisaged that this would lead to better utilisation of resources, better integrated and more streamlined clinical processes and improved quality of care for patients. Similar changes were being introduced in the health services of other countries, resulting from the recognition that healthcare has in recent times become increasingly complex and structures need to be put in place to support those people in similar specialties to work together and take collective responsibility for maximising resources to provide quality clinical care. Prior to this initiative, this responsibility would have rested primarily in the domain of the manager, who had the unenviable task of struggling to stay within budget while trying to meet the demands of individual clinicians for more resources and ensure that the best care is provided for all patients. CIM's aim was to delegate more of the decision making to clinicians so that these conflicting demands might be considered realistically.

Although the overall aims of the initiative were clearly communicated, the details of implementing it in individual hospitals was considered to be a matter for each hospital, with the recognition that imposing the same structure and processes for involving clinicians on all would not work. The Office for Health Management (OHM) played a key role in supporting the implementation of this initiative through workshops and training, and the provision of information and guidelines in the form of discussion papers and newsletters.

In 2000, the OHM conducted a review of the progress of CIM with the aim of sharing learning and experiences across the hospital sites and identifying what further support was needed by individual hospitals. Thirty-one hospitals throughout Ireland were visited as part of this review process.

This review identified that there was a sense of CIM being a centrally driven initiative (i.e. emanating from the Department of Health and Children) that had not made clear what the benefits would be at local level. Because of this there was little understanding of how the initiative should be implemented, although people did understand the broad aims. None of the hospitals that were reviewed had dedicated personnel at senior level charged with progressing the initiative. Because CIM was perceived as driven by managers it tended to focus on issues that are within the managers' domains – structures, resources, communication and service planning – with little discussion about the quality of clinical care.

cont/d

The Managers

Hospital managers seemed convinced of the merits of CIM but the reality of their daily lives, with increasing pressures, meant that few had been able to prioritise the implementation of CIM, with the result that very few sites had developed detailed implementation plans.

The Nurses

Nurses showed divided reactions to CIM. Some perceived it as changing the organisational structure and therefore changing the roles of nurses in senior positions. They were concerned about the devolution of management responsibility to integrated management units and the subsequent loss of the nursing hierarchy. On the other hand, there were nurses who were enthusiastic about CIM and perceived it as an opportunity for nurses to become more involved in multi-disciplinary working teams at unit level.

The Doctors

The involvement of doctors in CIM varied greatly across the thirty-one sites, with some having no involvement and others being very actively involved, leading integrated management units and working with a nurse manager and business manager. The review identified that in some cases low levels of involvement were indication of lack of interest but in others the lack of time to take on additional responsibilities was the primary problem. Many doctors are waiting for firm evidence that CIM benefited patients. In sites where there is an enthusiastic senior doctor committed to CIM more progress was observed.

The Therapeutic and Diagnostic Professions

In general the reaction of these professionals was a sense of threat. They feared the fragmentation of their professional departments that they believed would ensue from the re-structuring of hospitals into integrated management units. They were also concerned that they would have little influence at hospital level if CIM were fully implemented, as most of the attention was focused on involving doctors and nurses.

Questions

Reflecting on what you have read about large system change in this chapter, how would you explain the slow progress of the CIM?

1. Referring back to the Burke-Litwin model in chapter 4, identify the transformational factors that need to be addressed to revitalise the CIM initiative?

cont/d

2. Referring back to the Levels and Interlevels of chapter 5, describe an intervention:
   a) At the individual level, that would facilitate greater involvement of the doctors in this initiative.
   b) At the group level, that would address the sense of threat of the therapeutic and diagnostic professions.
   c) At the inter-group level, to engage the nurses, doctors and other professions in a team approach to progressing this initiative.

Note: The material for this case study was developed from one of the authors' involvement in some of the training and review of the CIM and from the OHM discussion paper on the findings of the review (OHM, 2001).

Clinical Inquiry Exercise 7.1

Think of a change process with which you are familiar.

Step 1   What are the external forces driving change?
         What are the internal forces driving change?
         How powerful are these forces?
         What choices do we have?

Step 2   If things keep going the way they are without significant intervention:
         What will be the predicted outcome?
         What is our desired outcome?

Step 3   What is it in the present that we need to change in order to get to our desired future – what is done, how work is done, structures, attitudes, culture…?

Step 4   What are the main avenues that will get us from here to there?
         What are the particular projects within those avenues? Long, medium, short term…
         How do we involve the organisation in this project?
         Where do we begin?
         What actions do we take to effect maximum effect? Medium effect?
         Minimum effect?
         How will we manage the transition?
         How do we build commitment? Who is/who is not ready/capable for change? How will we manage resistance?
         Who will let it happen, help it happen, make it happen?
         Do we need additional help – consultants, facilitators…?

Step 5   What review procedures do we need to establish?
         How do we articulate and share what we are learning?

CHAPTER 8

Working with Resistance to Change

Resistance to change is usually perceived as a disruptive force that needs to be overcome in order to move the organisation forward. It is a label applied by managers and consultants to the perceived behaviour of organisational members who seem unwilling to accept or implement an organisational change. It is typically used by those who are agents of a change and tends not be used by those who are the targets of the label to describe themselves.

Returning to Lewin we can say that any change process is typically conceived of having three stages – becoming motivated to change, changing what has been identified as needing to change, and making the change survive and work. These stages have been developed and given some specific elaboration by Schein (1980, 1999a). In the Lewin-Schein model, the creation of the motivation to change occurs through three processes. The first process is disconfirmation, in which present experiences tend to lead to frustration or dissatisfaction, as, for example, when goals or expectations are not met. As this information can be dismissed or ignored, in order that change may happen, the disconfirming information has to be accepted as valid and linked to something about which the system is concerned. The second process is the resultant anxiety or guilt which accompanies disconfirmation. Schein (1999a) refers to this as "survival anxiety", meaning that if there is no response to the disconfirming information, then some important elements of the system will fail. Schein makes the point that "survival anxiety" alone does not suffice for change to take place. A system can be blocked by what Schein calls "learning anxiety", which is that form of anxiety which promotes defensiveness, resistance and paralysis. A person may experience learning anxiety from the pain of unlearning, from feeling temporarily incompetent, a fear of losing one's identity or losing team membership or a fear of being punished. Increasing such learning anxiety has the effect of increasing paralysis and resistance.

Rashford and Coghlan (1994) added a further elaboration to Schein's disconfirmation process. The more unexpected the disconfirming information is, the more likely it is to be denied. The need for change is disputed as denial involves the rejection of the change information as not being relevant or pertinent. The dodging stage begins when the accumulated evidence shows that the change can no longer be denied and is likely to take place. It is then acknowledged reluctantly that some change is needed but that the change is required in other parts of the system – the "others have to change" response. Individuals and teams can seek ways to avoid or postpone change or remain peripheral to it.

It is at the dodging stage when passive-aggressive behaviour is more typical (McIlduff and Coghlan, 2000). Anger is directed at change agents – "those who are making me change". If an individual experiences the culture of the organisation as not supporting direct expression of anger and opposition, then passive-aggressive behaviours may follow, during which time individuals will not participate actively in change programmes. They may physically attend meetings and training events but do not "participate", and in their passivity communicate unexpressed hostility and opposition. At the same time they vent their opposition and lack of support to peers and friends outside of formal organisational situations. Coghlan and Rashford (1990) pointed to ways in which alienated members engage in distorted and faulty thinking about managerial behaviour. This means that individuals and teams, when they feel under threat, tend to over-generalise, deny the positive, be selective in what they perceive, jump to conclusions and act on the basis of emotional reasoning.

In times of change in organisations the psychological relationship between management and employees becomes more critical because it is in the context of change that management's expectations of the individual member and the individual member's expectations of management become more demanding. As Rashford and Coghlan (1994) point out, the bonding relationship between an individual and an organisation can come under pressure as a result of a change process. The way the change is introduced and managed can affect the individual's relationship to the changing or changed organisation, either positively or negatively.

Coercion to change without rationale, explanation or dialogue contributes to the development of stress from the sense of threat, ambiguity, powerlessness, isolation and overload, and leads to individual insecurity, anxiety, emotional exhaustion, alienation and demotivation (Ashforth and Lee, 1990).

The Process of Demotivation

Meyer (1977) reflects that people generally come to a job already motivated and that they are set on the road to demotivation by thoughtlessness and neglect. She describes six stages of demotivation. Stage 1 is the *Confusion* stage, where productivity drops slightly and the employee is wondering whether it is the boss or himself who is at fault. Stage 2 is the *Anger* stage where the employee's attitude becomes less positive and more angry as he tries to get the boss to notice that he is angry so that the boss will do something. Stage 3 is the *Subconscious*

Hope stage where there is no longer any doubt as to who is at fault and the employee tends to avoid the boss and withholds information. Stage 4 is the *Disillusionment* stage where the employee gives up taking any initiative and only does the basic job. Stage 5 is the *Uncooperative* stage where the employee refuses to do anything that is not clearly part of his job. Stage 6 is the *Final* stage where the employee either leaves the job or accepts it as a plodding eight hours to be filled.

The options for any individual who finds himself at Stage 6 of Meyer's Six Stages of Demotivation are to leave the organisation, sit on the fence, work the system, grumble persistently, find a niche, withdraw inwardly or create a neurotic mechanism (Merry and Brown, 1987). Leaving may not be a viable option, particularly in an economic recession, so the disillusioned employee may opt to work the system, which is to stay in the organisation and exploit it as best as possible for his own self-interest – securing all the benefits available, avoiding all volunteering and extra work, and managing to spend as little time as possible doing anything significant. Persistent grumbling is where the individual always complains and grumbles about conditions and how things are in the organisation. Some individuals manage to find a niche for themselves in which they create their own private enclave and reduce interdependence with others. Ashforth and Lee (1990) describe defensive behaviour as avoiding action by over-conforming, passing the buck, playing dumb, depersonalising, and stalling and avoiding blame by playing safe, justifying and scapegoating. The final option is to collaborate with others who feel the same as they do in creating a collective delusion, which in Merry and Brown's (1987) view becomes a neurotic mechanism. So there is blaming, hostility, aggression, anger, feelings of frustration and dysfunctional organisational behaviour that bind people into a collective delusion and serve to relieve the organisation of responsibility for confronting and dealing with its problems.

What are the dynamics of the change process for those who are being mandated to change by their managers? For individuals, teams and the interdepartmental group, there are three critical process elements (Coghlan, 2000b). These are:

1. *Perception of the change.* This comprises the meaning the change has for them, the degree to which they have control over the change and the degree of trust in those promoting the change.
2. *Assessment of the impact of the change.* Participants may assess the perceived impact of the change along a continuum, ranging from positively enhancing at one extreme, through uncertain to threatening or destructive at the other.
3. *Response.* The individual can deny, dodge, oppose, resist, tolerate, accept, support or embrace the change.

These three elements are influenced heavily by the availability of information about the change and the process of communication between those promoting the change and those affected by it. Absence of information and a lack of a sense of participation create anxiety, uncertainty, hesitation and resistance, thereby increasing any lack of trust that might exist.

For a large system to change, key individuals have to be motivated to change and have to have done something about what needs changing. Key teams have to apply themselves to the change, the change must be generalised at the interdepartmental group level and the organisation must adapt in its external markets (Rashford and Coghlan, 1994). Any organisational change processes involve individuals, teams and groups reacting to the change and responding in the light of their perception of what they think it means for them. There are extensive meetings of individuals and teams to share information, solve problems and make decisions. Frequently, there are negotiations for resources by inter-functional teams at the interdepartmental group level. All these activities occur in order to move the organisation from a stage of disconfirming information to a renewed state. Accordingly, the change process comprises a series of movements, as individuals and teams deal with the change issues and negotiate them with other individuals and teams.

SOURCES OF INDIVIDUAL RESISTANCE TO ORGANISATIONAL CHANGE

Watson (1969: 488) defines resistance as "all forces which contribute to stability in personality or social systems". Zaltman and Duncan (1977: 63) provide a similar definition. "We define resistance here as any conduct that serves to maintain the status quo in the face of pressure to alter the status quo". In their view, resistance may be caused by the change agents and may be justifiable in cases where the change may be harmful to individuals or to a group. It is useful to remember that every change involves some form of loss and letting go something that is familiar. Change requires going from the known to the unknown, and so dissolves meaning and challenges assumptions that an individual has built up about himself/herself (Tannenbaum and Hanna, 1985).

What then are the sources of resistance to organisational change? Kotter and Schlesinger (1979) list the common sources: parochial self-interest, misunderstanding and lack of trust, different assessments of what change is required and a low tolerance for change. An examination of their list shows that, in their view, the sources of resistance exist in both the personality and the situation. Hussey (1995) identifies a range of factors that might explain the causes of resistance:

- *Actual threats*: changes that are perceived as having an impact on the value of an individual's job generally tend to raise fears and uncertainties.
- *Imposed change*: if individuals do not understand why changes are imposed on them they will tend to resist them.
- *Lack of faith in those making the change*: this usually comes about when people have previous experience of the change agent(s) inability to manage change.
- *The head and the heart*: individuals may intellectually agree that change is required, but emotionally be happier to maintain the status quo.

There are numerous forces in individuals that limit their ability and willingness to participate in change (Watson, 1969; Neumann, 1989). Change is hard because it upsets the comfort of the present. Even though the present situation might have its difficulties, at least it is familiar; the devil you know is better than the devil you don't know. It is difficult to change habits. People get used to working and thinking in a certain way and when they have to change it takes a lot of concentration and energy. It is so easy to slip back into the old ways. They tend to have a preferred way of solving problems. They tend to manage their conflicts in much the same way. Whatever ways they have learned over the years they tend to stick with – opt out/fight back aggressively/be dismissive/sulk... If they are stuck in one form of reaction then that limits their ability to select the appropriate response.

One of biggest problems people have is that they tend to see things from their own point of view only. They can be biased, prejudiced and ignorant of other valid viewpoints. They can stereotype others, attribute motivations and project their own fantasies onto others. Their upbringing can hold them back. Some were reared or professionally trained not to stand up for themselves, to always say "yes" or to think conservatively. Some people can get into feeling helpless, that they have no power. This comes with the notion that there is a powerful "they" who is doing all this, and so individuals can distort reality by thinking that this powerful "they" has all the power and individuals have none. A further distortion is a form of self-distrust, where some people undermine their own self-confidence and their self-respect. It is in this regard that assertiveness training and personal development courses are useful in enabling people deal with change. Some find that when they think about asserting themselves and getting in touch with how they feel and what they want, they are pulled back by all sorts of taboos. There are tapes in their head telling them not to push themselves forward, that they should be nice to people, that they should not cause upset... Some find that when they are under threat and the present and future are uncertain they can easily find themselves looking to the past and hankering after the "good old days", even though we all know that these "good old days" were anything but good. Regressing into the past is a way of avoiding the challenge of the present and future.

Sources of resistance to change can also be found in the situation, that is to say that a cause of resistance is found in how the change is being managed or communicated (Quirke, 1996). Examples of situational sources of resistance to change are when management fails to be specific about a change, to show why change is necessary or to give those affected by the change a say in the planning of the process. As we have seen, when management fails to allay fears and worries about job security or to keep employees informed as to what is happening and disregards work-habit patterns, employees are more likely to respond negatively or critically to a change programme. Other situational sources of resistance can be a lack of trust, the culture of the organisation, adversarial relations and polarisation of positions.

When we inquire further into the twin sources of individual resistance to change, individual and situational, we find that situational sources are the most common. That is to say, most resistance to change is actually caused by management behaviour – lack of information, lack of consultation and so on. Yet, it is the individual's personality which is most commonly targeted. An individual is not flexible or is a traditionalist. This shows us how resistance is typically presented as a position on change from the perspective of those who are actually promoting the change. Klein (1969) takes the position of the defender and argues for a sensitivity towards the issues that the resisters present. In his view those resisting change rarely define themselves as such; they see themselves as defending something they think will be lost. In a similar vein, Nevis (1987) makes the point that people resisting change in an organisation are frequently high-powered members and that resistance is a creative source of energy. In his view, resistance has meaning only in the context of a power differential. Those with less power cannot easily say no to those with greater power. Accordingly, those with less power who are saying no are perceived as being resistant, much like a child saying no to a parent is perceived. The key solution, in Nevis' view, is in how managerial authority and power are conceived and the role dissent, debate and disagreement play in the dissemination of power and influence in decision making. Nevis also cautions against viewing resistance in terms of the emotional element only and emphasises that the cognitive element should be also taken into account. Resistance can be a healthy response to change and is often an indication of a flaw in the planned change. It can serve as a trigger that leads to re-examination of the plans and a resultant improvement in the change process, or it can lead to the change agents stubbornly maintaining their course and risking escalated resistance and entrenched positions on both sides.

RESISTANCE TO CHANGE IN GROUPS AND TEAMS

It is clear that membership of an organisation typically involves membership of groups and teams: a) face-to-face working teams in the formal structures of the organisation, b) participation on committees, temporary task forces, c) membership of a professional association or trade union and d) participation in informal groups of colleagues/peers with whom we associate and which help shape our perceptions and attitudes. Reactions and responses to change are often shaped by the groups in which we work and with which we identify.

Group Norms and Culture

When groups/teams form and are together for a period they typically settle into patterns of behaving, thinking and relating. Habits grow up around such elements as: how things get done, how to relate to authority, who socialises with whom, how influence is exerted, how time is used, how successes and failures are dealt with and so on. These patterns become the group's "unwritten rules" and they frequently constitute what we would call the "atmosphere" or "climate" in a group or team. Nurses notice the difference between working in one hospital or community care area and another, one ward or health centre and another, one specialised unit and another. This difference is often intangible and hard to describe. It is partly about atmosphere and mostly about established traditions around the important issues of working and relating. Informal rules are in place which help keep the group "unique" and help survival of the group.

When the group takes on new members they are socialised into the group's patterns of behaving and thinking. The new member learns the ropes and learns how to get on in this group. If a new member unwittingly breaks one of the "informal rules", he/she can be informed that, "We don't do that around here". Continuous breach of any of these rules that are judged to be important results in the new member being punished in some way and ultimately being expelled from the group: "She never fitted in; she wasn't our type."

A group's tradition can be handed on from generation to generation, even long after the original members have left, so that after a while the group is unaware that these "rules" exist and are influencing the group. The rules have disappeared from awareness because they have become taken for granted and no one notices them any more. At the same time they exert an influence on how the group functions. When it comes to issues of change, the deeply embedded traditions and assumptions that are held by the members play a key role in how change is facilitated or resisted (Schein, 1999a). Individual health professionals tend to have strong group norms and profession-specific cultures. For example, in the medical profession there is the norm of working long hours as a junior doctor or the expectation that the medically qualified person will be the automatic leader of any multidisciplinary group. These professional norms and cultures are reinforced by other professions' perceptions and resulting behaviour. For example, nurses defer to doctors because they believe that is what is expected.

Groups and Change

The central research with regard to groups and change was conducted by Kurt Lewin (1948). Lewin found that when a group as a whole made a decision to have its members change their behaviour it was more effective in producing actual change than a series of lectures from outsiders that provided information and exhorted change. One of Lewin's close associates, Cartwright, has drawn together much of the research on how groups function in relation to change (Cartwright, 1989). As a source of influence on their members, groups are a significant medium of change. The chances of change seem to be increased when a group's members have a strong sense of belonging to the same group. The more attractive the group is to its members the greater the influence the group can exert over its members. In attempts to change attitudes, values and behaviour the more relevant the values, attitudes and behaviours are to the basis of attraction to the group the greater influence the group can exert on them, as instanced when a union executive seeks support for action on issues of conditions of employment. The greater the prestige of a group member in the eyes of other members the greater the influence he/she can exert. Efforts to change individuals/sub-parts of a group, which if successful would result in making them deviate from the group norms, will encounter resistance.

Sources of Resistance to Changes in Groups and Teams

Zaltman and Duncan (1977) describe five ways in which teams function to resist change:

1. *Team solidarity.* This can bind members together in a way that resists a change that would break up the team or affect the relationships within it. The evidence connecting team cohesiveness to the likelihood of resistance is mixed. Some studies found that more cohesive teams react more favourably to change, provided it does not threaten to break up the team, while non-cohesive teams are very threatened because they do not have a framework for mutual support. On the other hand, cohesive teams can be very resistant because of the close identification among the members.
2. *Rejection of outsiders.* When there is a high degree of in-group

identification change that is initiated from outside the team is resisted.

3. *Conformity to norms.* As already described above, a group's norms and culture may be so deeply embedded that change threatens its stability and is incompatible with these norms and so is resisted.

4. *Conflict.* In an inter-group conflict situation what is accepted by one group may be rejected automatically by other groups.

5. *Team insight.* If a group or team has not participated in any teambuilding, formal or informal, which has helped to create a sense of group or team, its members may lack the ability to reflect on what is happening and have no collective frame of reference with which to evaluate a proposed change.

Inter-group Dynamics

The dynamics of inter-team conflict are well-documented (Schein, 1980). Groups in conflict develop uniform, stereotyped views of themselves and those with whom they are in conflict. These views are evident in selective perceptions of the best in one's own position, denying its own weaknesses, and perceiving only the worst parts of the other team, tending to deny its strengths, and developing a negative stereotype of the other team. These positions have an effect on communication between the teams as each team tends to listen only to its own representative and to accept only what confirms the stereotyped perceptions.

A change process frequently involves inter-team conflict in organisational settings where the change is promoted by a management/administration group and those affected by the change feel apart from that group and oppose the change. In such situations, groups can bond together in opposition to other groups and so begins the process of selective perceptions, distortions and stereotyping of the other groups. Communication becomes difficult and it is not uncommon to require a mediator or third party to facilitate communication and resolution of the conflict.

In the cognitive mode, Argyris (1990) grounds resistance to change in the psychological structure of organisations low in openness, trust and risk-taking, and high in conformity and mistrust from which carefully built and brilliantly concealed defensive routines are created. As managers propagate and build systems to maintain these defensive routines, the propensity to resist change is increased.

BARRIERS TO CHANGE IN HEALTHCARE

There are particular characteristics of healthcare environments that make them susceptible to certain common types of barriers to change as outlined below:

Autonomy Expectations of Health Professionals

The nature of healthcare is such that the work has a high level of importance as it involves personal and highly critical matters of human suffering and life-and-death issues. A complex technology and knowledge base is required for much of the work and as a result health professionals have traditionally been afforded a high level of professional autonomy and functional independence in their work. This leads to resistance to attempts to introduce any formal methods of monitoring or assessing the quality of care, as it can threaten their autonomy.

Collective Benefits of Stability

Healthcare environments tend to be highly routinised with standard operating procedures, mandatory communication patterns etc. There are perceived benefits to maintaining routine and stability, and any attempt to change such routines are likely to meet with resistance. A typical example is the practice of early breakfast for patients to ensure that everything is ready for the ward round. In reality ward rounds may not take place until late morning, the patients having been served breakfast at 6.30/7 a.m. Changing this routine would probably benefit many patients, but in the short term would create instability in the work patterns of staff and is therefore resisted by some.

Calculated Opposition to Change

Change usually results in a shift in the power balance and may result in the loss of power, status and influence for some. Those who perceive change as depriving them of their prevailing advantage will resist the change. For example, some clinicians resist others' attempts to involve them in the management of services, as they perceive such a move as reducing their power to use resources autonomously without regard for the impact on other services.

Tunnel Vision

Health professionals can become so concentrated in their specialised functions (particularly as healthcare is rapidly developing more and more subspecialties) that individuals tend to lose sight of the bigger picture and broader possibilities of change and innovation. This can result in a situation where only incremental or small-scale change is acceptable.

Resource Limitations

Limited financial resources and acute shortages of personnel can mean that staff get locked into established behaviours and do not take the time to reflect and improve work practices. They therefore become powerless to create change. This manifests itself in staff who cannot find time to attend the project meetings for a change initiative.

Sunk Costs

Resources are allocated to specific projects and there is no pool of finances to implement change projects across the system. Many investments are not convertible and do not translate into perceived tangible benefits such as increased throughput, reduced lengths of stay or reduced waiting lists. This makes it difficult to justify investments in projects such as installing new information systems.

Unofficial and Unplanned Constraints on Behaviour

The healthcare environment has many informal organisations within it. These can wield significant power (e.g. the power of the unions to call for strikes or work stoppages) and can slow the process of change by a variety of subtle, but effective strategies and actions.

WORKING WITH RESISTANCE

We are taking the approach that resistance is something to be worked with, rather than something to be overcome. "Overcoming" resistance tends to imply a coercive approach and such an approach is likely to lead to increased resistance and opposition (Nevis, 1987; Goldstein, 1989). The OD approach to resistance is to treat it with respect by considering it as a healthy, self-regulating manifestation that must be taken seriously.

The most common OD guidelines for working with resistance are: involve people in the planning of change, provide accurate and complete information, give employees an opportunity to air their objections, provide adequate motivation (make explicit the benefits to all), develop a trusting climate, take organisational culture into consideration and use problem-solving approaches. Kotter and Schlesinger (1979) outline a number of approaches (education, participation, facilitation, negotiation, manipulation and coercion) and show in what situations they are commonly used, as well as the advantages and disadvantages of each approach. Education is a useful approach when communicating a change to a large number of people who ought to know about the change but may not be directly affected by it. An example is where a hospital is planning to change its name and introduce a new logo. Not all staff needs to be involved in the process of change, but all should know about the change and understand the reasons for it and what the new logo signifies. Participation is a useful approach when a change is widespread and has implications for everyone in the organisation. For example, if a community care area is introducing a quality accreditation system there should be participation by all groups of staff in determining how best to implement the system. Facilitation is the most appropriate approach for implementing change in a team or department where the emphasis needs to be on problem solving. For example, a social-work team wants to review its waiting list and reach agreement on a new system for managing the waiting list. An external facilitator is invited in to help the team identify problems and possible solutions. Negotiation may be the most appropriate approach when groups hold fairly entrenched positions on an issue. For example, if clerks are demanding more pay for implementing a new patient record system that has already been designed and installed, management may need to negotiate the change and agree changes in conditions. Manipulation and coercion may be approaches that, though undesirable, are necessary in crisis situations.

A common theme or issue that emerges in situations of resistance is poor communication "We weren't told", "Why are we only hearing about this now". Although every change agent and manager knows the importance of communication, it remains one of the central difficulties in the change process. The difficulty arises not because there is no communication but because insufficient thought is given to how and what to communicate. A good communicator starts from the question "What is it the audience or recipients of the communication are most likely to want to know?" whereas the more common approach is starting from "What are the good/positive things I can tell them about?" "What must we not tell them about?" "What should I leave out because it might only result in negativity and resistance?" Qualified communication, although useful in some situations (e.g. when trying to prevent the entire workforce walking out), almost invariably results in the audience/recipients feeling that their intelligence has been underestimated, and this can be a powerful motivator for resisting change. Resistance if met with defensiveness and an unwillingness to change the plan will become more entrenched. Openness and ongoing sharing and communication, coupled with a flexible approach to implementing the change are the key ingredients in preventing pockets of entrenched resistance developing in an organisation.

CONCLUSIONS

In this chapter we have mapped out the kinds of things that tend to happen when change is not managed properly. If staff are not involved in a change process, not consulted and do not feel any sense of meaningful participation, they become demotivated, alienated and tend to move towards dysfunctional behaviour and resist the change. Such dysfunctional behaviour has a negative effect on the organisation's work and has a cumulative effect on the people concerned. Change makes demands on people that can be threatening, create stress and generate anxiety. If these feelings are added to by uncertainty, confusion, anger and bitterness then one would expect individuals to go into some sort of self-protection mode and so the central organisational issues of how to change become very secondary.

People become demotivated and alienated when they feel they are not listened to and when their experience and commitment are not being valued. Such a sense of lack of consideration exists because there is actually a lack of consideration on management's behalf or it can exist because management does not know how to consult, show appreciation or create commitment to change. Inadequacies at the management level in this regard actually create a significant proportion of problems in change.

It is becoming increasingly evident that organisations not only need to change, but in doing so learn how to change and learn how to learn about change. A core element of such a learning process is to study the effect of mismanaged change on staff and understand how such consequences have come about, and how they could be avoided for the future.

In summary:

- Resistance is a natural phenomenon; it is an essential element in understanding change.
- Resistance to change has it origins in the personality and the situation. The personality is typically cited as the cause of resistance, while resistance is commonly caused by the situation.
- Resistance is not passive but is rather a dynamic energy.
- Resistance has both a cognitive and an emotional element.
- There are differing degrees of acceptance to change and resistance to it – from enthusiastic acceptance and cooperation through passive resignation, indifference, apathy, passive resistance to active and open opposition.
- Resistance is viewed generally from the perspective of those promoting change and there is a need to understand the perspective of the defenders.
- Resistance should be taken seriously, by being listened to, understood and acted on; it is an occasion for the change agents to look again at the change project, review omissions or errors and modify the project in the light of feedback.

Case 8.1 Cinicians in Management Initiative, Part B

Ann Reynolds is a clinical nurse manager responsible for the surgical ward in St Michael's. Before leaving for work one morning she was glancing through the morning paper and noticed an article on the launch of the "Clinicians in Management" (CIM) initiative. She read it with interest, thought the idea of involving clinicians in the management of hospitals made sense and wondered why nothing had been mentioned about this in St Michaels. That day she asked a number of her colleagues and one of the surgeons if they had heard anything about it, but nobody had. Ann put it to the back of her mind.

Three months later at a meeting between the ward managers and director of nursing, the director announced that the hospital was piloting a CIM structure in part of the hospital. Cardio-thoracic specialties would become an integrated management unit, as the hospital was a national centre for this area. All other surgery would form a second management unit. Each of the units would be managed by a consultant and a nurse manager. Ann's first thought was how her ward would be affected. Would her ward be split in two? Would she have to separate all records and accounts as if she was managing two wards? These issues were unclear for her. She spoke to a consultant after the meeting who said "of course this is their [management's] way of watching what we are spending and introducing more cutbacks – patient care is at the bottom of the list as usual. They've started with us because they think we waste more resources than anyone else. Next they will be asking us to sterilise our own equipment."

Later that day when Ann was in her office, another consultant dropped in to see how one of his post-op patients was doing and mentioned to Ann that he was enthusiastic that they might "finally get some resources around here and have an opportunity to let management know the real problems we face". Ann began to wonder what was going on. She went to the director of nursing and asked what CIM was meant to do for the hospital. The director explained that the purpose was to involve clinicians in decision making and this would hopefully lead to less resource wastage as well as better patient care. Ann later spoke to one of her colleagues in the Intensive Care Unit (ICU) who said that all the nursing staff in ICU were totally against this as they felt the existing situation was OK and this change would not only result in the consultants meddling in nursing issues, but the nurse managers of these units would create an additional layer between ward managers and the director of nursing. She pointed out the fiasco when the hospital had appointed a deputy director of nursing two years previously (she resigned after three months complaining that she could not do her job if she was not kept informed

cont/d

about what was happening at ward level). Ann's colleague told her that having had a number of informal meetings on this the nurses were of the unanimous opinion that publicly they should go along with this plan, as they believed they were powerless to stop it happening. They would, however, continue to report only to the Director of Nursing and would not give any information to the ward manager, who was likely to be an "outsider" in any case.

Questions

1. What do you think Ann will do?
2. Analyse the factors contributing to resistance at individual, group and inter-group levels within St Michael's hospital.
3. Refer back to chapter 7 and factor into your overall implementation plan a strategy to deal with the resistance that is emerging in this case.

Clinical Inquiry Exercise 8.1

Reflect on a change situation with which you are familiar.

1. Was the proposed change well explained?
2. Did organisational members have an input into what was to change and how?
3. Were there opposition, hesitancy and anxiety about the proposed change?
4. What was the basis for this opposition, hesitancy and anxiety?
5. How were the opposition, hesitancy and anxiety handled?
6. What were the outcomes in terms of a) effective implementation of change and b) the longer residue of feelings and morale in the organisation?
7. From this situation what have you learned about change that you would want to a) repeat in the future and b) avoid in the future?

CHAPTER 9

Leading Change in Organisations

The literature on leadership of organisations is vast and disparate. Leadership needs to be distinguished from authority and management. In chapter 4 we noted the comparison between management and leadership. Definitions of leadership range from the concept of giving a sense of direction – "Leadership is about a sense of direction ... It's knowing what the next step is" (Adair, 1990: 58) – to the concept of a process – "Leadership is a process whereby an individual influences a group of individuals to achieve a common goal" (Northouse, 1997: 3).

Early definitions of leadership focused on personality characteristics and traits, values and beliefs. However, it soon became obvious that it was not possible to predict characteristics or traits that would work in all situations. Also research began to show that other factors could have a stronger influence or relationship with organisational change. For example, Mohr's (1969) study of health officers found that leader values were more directly related to change and innovation in organisations where there were plentiful resources than in organisations with scarce resources. Also in Kimberly and Evanisko's (1981) study of American hospitals, some aspects of the organisational structures proved to be better predictors of ability to change and innovate than the leader's traits or characteristics.

Research subsequently shifted towards a quest for the leadership styles and leadership behaviour required for successful change management. The Ohio State University leadership studies (as well as a wide range of studies) that used the Ohio framework is the most widely known example of the leadership-style approach. They identified a dichotomy, which is still popular, between employee-centred and job-centred leadership. Two concepts were identified as being important in leadership – "Initiating Structure" and "Consideration". Initiating Structure is the extent to which a leader is likely to define and structure his own role and that of subordinates and provide clear definitions of role responsibility in goal attainment (emphasis is on the task). The second concept, consideration, is the extent to which a leader is likely to have job relationships that are characterised by mutual trust, respect for subordinates' ideas, regard for their feelings and open two-way communication. These studies have subsequently been criticised for failing to take situational variables into account (Korman, 1966).

The importance of vision, participatory rather than autocratic style and a democratic approach to change began to emerge as key features in successful American companies, views supported by Peters and Waterman (1982) and Kanter (1983). Since the late 1980s this notion of one best leadership style has been criticised. Writers such as Dunphy and Stace, (1990) argue that a contingency approach explains leadership, in that a particular style of leadership may be appropriate depending on organisational conditions, i.e. culture, climate, openness, trust and organisational members' attitudes towards change. King and Anderson (1995: 97) argue that evidence from "real-world studies" support the view that "where an organisation faces a threatening, turbulent environment, with members who are suspicious of change, leaders may need to be authoritarian rather than participative in order to implement innovations".

One of the more important works on leadership is Burns' classic (1978) distinction between transactional and transformational leaders. We have already seen this distinction in the dimensions of the Burke-Litwin model. Transactional leadership emphasises the transaction that takes place between the leader and the subordinate in any situation. This type of leadership occurs when a leader takes the initiative and offers some form of need satisfaction (pay, promotion, recognition) in response for performance. The transactional leader sets clear goals, understands the needs of employees and selects appropriate, motivating rewards. The approach emphasises the importance of the relationship between a leader and his/her followers, focusing on the mutual benefits arising from the "transaction". Transformational leadership involves the use of charisma to transform a vision into shared objectives. Burns contends that transformational leadership involves the maximum amount of mutual trust and the minimum amount of coercion. The leader goes beyond the norm to bring about change in the attitudes and behaviour of followers and in the process helps followers identify their full potential.

Bass and Avolia (1994) define transformational leadership as something that occurs when leaders:

- Stimulate interest among colleagues and followers to view their work from new perspectives.
- Generate awareness of the mission or vision of the team and organisation.
- Develop colleagues and followers to higher levels of leadership and potential.
- Motivate colleagues and followers to look beyond their own interests towards those that will benefit the group.

Transformational leadership is a process for engaging the commitment of staff to a shared vision and shared values. It is a form of leadership that is particularly important in leading change, as it involves a relationship of mutual trust between leader and followers. According to Bass and Avolia (1994), transactional and transformational leadership have been observed to varying degrees in healthcare organisations. They argue that transformational leadership is an extension of transactional leadership, rather than a separate dimension. In a study of 71 middle managers in the Irish health services, using Bass and Avolia's Multifactor Leadership Questionnaire, Armstrong (1999) found that over half of the managers scored above the median on both transactional and transformational leadership. No respondent received a low score on transformational leadership. Carney (1999) argues the case that transformational leadership is the style best suited to nursing, as nurse managers are well placed to work in participative cooperation and to empower staff. McCarthy (1998), writing about leadership in nursing, expressed the view that very few transforming leaders had emerged in Irish nursing. She believes that Irish nurse leaders "in the main have been the products of autocratic systems and mentored into using primarily transactional roles" (1998: 240). More recently there has been a considerable effort to develop nursing leadership in Ireland through leadership development programmes, mentoring and learning sets.

Images of Leadership

The dominant image of leadership is the military one, which is not surprising given that armies and their leaders have been the major source of our experience of organisations over the centuries. So we use military terminology in talking about organisations – strategy, tactics, obeying orders, compliance – and sometimes refer to the business of the organisation as a battleground or as a war. Hierarchy and the chain of command in organisations largely developed from the military model. We may refer to those in the direct service of customers as "the troops", those "in the trenches" or "in the front line". This has all changed in recent years. We now see the "troops" as "knowledge workers". We see leadership, not in terms of command and control but in terms of empowerment, alignment and path finding.

Mintzberg (1998) takes the image of the conductor of an orchestra as an image for leadership. He illustrates how, far from the notion we tend to have of the conductor as an autocratic dictator, the conductor is a leader of professionals who work with little direction from a manager. Mintzberg notes that what we see as control of the orchestra (sitting in the same seats, playing the same notes, high degrees of coordination and so on) is a control that comes from the profession, rather than direction from the manager/conductor. Hence for Mintzberg, leadership of professionals is covert, rather than overt. The conductor is a leader among equals yet does not take the lead or set the pace. Mintzberg makes the connection with hospital surgeons and university professors who describe their structures as upside down with themselves at the top and managers below to serve them.

In an important edited volume on the leader of the future (Hesselbein, Goldsmith and Beckhard, 1996), some of the major writers on leadership – Stephen Covey, Peter Drucker, Charles Handy, James Kouzes, Barry Posner and Edgar Schein among others – explore what it means to lead the organisation of tomorrow, what skills, actions and strategies will be required and how leaders will need to develop. Repeated across these many writings are arguments for leaders to envision, empower, coach, serve, lead diversity and shape culture, for leaders to be learners themselves and to manage their own self-learning. In discussions on leadership there is a danger in focusing on the leader alone, as it tends to propagate the notion of the leader as hero. The reality is more complex. Leaders are leaders of systems, the dynamics of which enable or inhibit leaders to exercise their function.

THE LEADERSHIP GRID®

For people working in organisations the behaviour or style of leaders is what they experience most directly and is that which either energises or frustrates them most. Robert Blake and Jane Mouton developed a framework for understanding and evaluating human effectiveness and management over thirty years ago. This framework, originally called the Managerial Grid® and now the Leadership Grid®, has been refined and developed over that period (Blake and Mouton, 1964, 1978; Blake and McCanse, 1991; McKee and Carlson, 1999) and has been applied to nursing leadership (Blake, Mouton and Tapper, 1981) and to patient care (Prather, Blake and Mouton, 1990). In its essence, the Grid charts a range of behavioural choices along a three-dimensional figure. The horizontal axis shows a concern for outcome or results on a scale of 1 to 9. An individual leader may be high (a score of 9), low (a score of 1) or in the middle (a score of 5) on concern for outcome. On the vertical axis, which shows a concern for people on a scale of 1 to 9, an individual leader may be high (a score of 9), low (a score of 1) or in the middle (a score of 5) on concern for people. Putting these horizontal and vertical axes together gives a two-dimensional grid with seven points plotted on it (Figure 9.1). Each point may be viewed as a Grid style.

While the two concerns may be viewed as independent, they actually merge when forming a Grid style. When individuals work with others on a task, the concerns become interdependent. They may be compared to ingredients in making a cake. Ingredients, such as flour and sugar, exist

Figure 9.1 The Leadership Grid

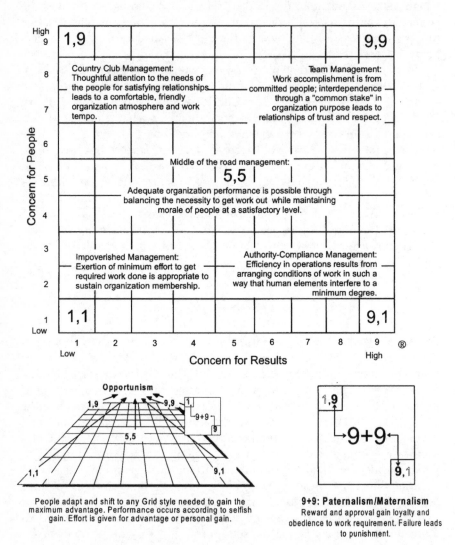

Source: The Leadership Grid® figure, Paternalism Figure and Opportunism from Leadership Dilemmas--Grid Solutions, by Robert R. Blake and Anne Adams MoCanse (Formerly the Managerial Grid by Robert R. Blake and Jane S. Mouton). Houston: Gulf Publishing Company (Grid Figure: P 29, Paternalism Figure: p. 30, Opportunism Figure: p. 31). Copyright 1991 by Scientific Methods, Inc. Reproduced by permission of the owners.

independently but in being mixed and baked, they merge to help form a cake. In Grid terms, this interdependence can be explained through the following example. If the following high concern for outcome, "I exert vigorous effort to achieve outcomes", stands alone it does not say much about how I work with others. However, if I say, "I exert vigorous effort to achieve outcomes and force others to comply" then I am illustrating that my high concern for outcomes (9) is joined by a low concern for people (1). On the other hand, my high concern for outcome may be "I exert vigorous effort to achieve outcomes and others work with me enthusiastically". In this instance, my high concern for outcome (9) is accompanied by a high concern for people (9).

There is a third dimension which is a motivational scale on which is plotted something of the range of reasons why people operate out of a particular Grid style, ranging from the "+" end of seeking something the leader wants or needs to the "-" end, which reflects something the leader wants to avoid. This third dimension provides a framework for reflecting on and understanding personal motivations.

9,1: Authority-Compliance

The 9,1 oriented style is located at the lower right hand corner of the Grid and marks a style that has a high concern for task with people's needs receiving low concern. Leaders' emphasis is on efficiency and results, with subordinates expected to carry out their commands. Why do 9,1 leaders act this way? At one extreme of the motivational scale is a desire for mastery and control and at the other a fear of failure. 9,1 oriented leaders control authorisation, are hard driving, distrustful, find fault and make all the decisions. Conflict is perceived as a threat to authority. For example, the newly appointed CEO of a hospital in his first meeting with his management team makes it explicit that his only concern is staying within budget and indicating that he will not accept any budget over-runs from his managers regardless of the circumstances. A month later he freezes recruitment, and issues a directive to discontinue all temporary contracts. When one of his managers indicates he is likely to exceed the budget, he insists that all expenditure for this programme must be counter-signed by him.

1,9: Country Club

The 1,9 oriented style is located at the top left hand corner of the Grid and marks a style that has a high concern for people and a low concern for task. 1,9 oriented leaders place a primary emphasis on creating a happy atmosphere where people's feelings and needs are catered for, with outcomes receiving a lower concern. Why do 1,9 oriented leaders act in this way? At one extreme 1,9 leaders desire to please and at the other there is a fear of rejection. They feel secure when relationships are positive and others are accepting and approving, while avoiding criticism because it means rejection and hurt. They cannot say No, are sensitive and easily hurt. Conflict is avoided because 1,9 oriented leaders take it personally.

Decision making is only "nice" when people embrace it and engage in sharing. For example, a newly appointed general manager suddenly has managerial responsibility for the team of which she was formerly a member. She has replaced a much disliked, authoritarian manager. She vows that she will put the welfare of her staff uppermost on her agenda. She is also concerned about how her former colleagues will perceive her. She really wants to be seen as a caring manager who listens to people's problems. Meetings with her team can last up to three hours (as she believes everyone should have the opportunity to contribute). Work piles up on her desk. She finds decisions difficult as she wants to make sure everyone is happy.

1,1: Impoverished

The 1,1 oriented leader style is located at the lower left hand corner of the Grid and marks a style where there is a low concern for task and a low concern for people. It is a style whereby individual leaders have opted out of responsibility. Why do 1,1 oriented leaders behave like this? At one extreme is the desire to remain uninvolved and at the other a fear of termination. 1,1 oriented leaders do not want the position and so are non-committal, avoid conflict and go through the motions. At the same time they hide their feelings of discontent and do not face up to their desires not to have the responsibility. Sometimes this style can be associated with ill health or impending retirement. For example, if a consultant paediatrician is appointed as director of a child and maternal health directorate, but is only interested in building a strong paediatric research team, she may give less priority to her duties as leader of the directorate. She may consider herself the director in name only, believing that her colleagues are capable of looking after their own clinical specialties. Thus she exhibits little interest in their activities or welfare and does not embrace the rationale for integrating specialties into a single directorate.

5,5: Middle of the Road

The 5,5 oriented Grid style is located at the centre of the Grid and marks a compromise position of balancing the two concerns. On the one hand, 5,5 oriented leaders are motivated by a desire to belong and on the other a fear of humiliation. Accordingly, they set a middle path of accommodation, not rocking the boat, going with the majority, following precedent and tradition and trying to keep everyone happy. This style of leadership is sometimes evident in leaders who have slowly worked their way up through the organisation, and obtained the leader's position by virtue of entitlement rather than ability. They typically are content to follow someone else's vision rather than develop their own.

9,9: Team

The 9,9 oriented Grid style is located at the top right hand corner of the Grid and marks an integrated high concern for task and for people, with which there is no contradiction. This does not mean that everyone gets what they want or that they agree with the final decision, but that they are involved in the process, feel heard, understand what is happening and why. Thus there is commitment. 9,9 oriented leaders are motivated by a desire for fulfilment through contribution on the one hand and on the other a fear of selfishness, which loses the contribution of others. 9,9 oriented leaders see conflict as good, as it brings the issues into the open so they can work to solve them directly with understanding and agreement. 9,9 oriented leaders build commitment around vision, standards of excellence, clear expectations, shared values, and participation in problem solving and decision making. This does not mean that everyone is always involved in every decision. The underlying principle is that each is responsible for his/her own actions and that people can learn from reflecting on experience. Kieran (1998) studied the role of culture in the relationship between the statutory and voluntary sectors in disability services in Ireland. He adapted Blake and Mouton's grid to look at preferred and perceived cultural orientation in each sector. Both sectors agreed that 9,9, orientation culture, which assumes no inherent contradiction between the organisation's purpose and the needs of people, is the most productive. The voluntary sector were perceived by the statutory sector and rated themselves as operating according to this 9,9 style. By contrast the statutory sector were perceived by the voluntary sector and rated themselves as operating within a 9,1 style, i.e. having a low concern for people and a high concern for production and obedient performance.

9+9: Paternalist/Maternalist

The 9+9 oriented Grid style is a combination of 1,9 and 9,1, where there is a simultaneous high concern for task and people but they are not integrated. Paternalism or maternalism portrays behaviour from the two styles in a way that utilises reward and punishment. The high 9 of concern for people is contingent on the other person's compliance and support. Paternalistic leaders are parental figures, benevolent autocrats, dispensing approval and disapproval, and demanding loyalty. Why do 9+9 oriented leaders act in this way? At one extreme there is the desire for veneration and at the other the fear of repudiation. Paternalistic leaders enjoy admiration, giving advice and approval, and having others emulate them as models. They are hurt when their advice is ignored and are blind to any smothering effect their behaviour might be having. They may induce guilt through condescending behaviour which stunts growth in others. They are the sole decision maker and decisions are made for the good of others.

Any consultation is an illusion. A typical example is a ward manager who rewards people that are loyal by ensuring they get weekends off, whilst ensuring that poor performers or nurses who challenge her authority are scheduled to work weekends. However, this arrangement only works as long as loyalty and good performance are evident. If the loyal nurse makes one mistake she will be punished just like the challengers. Such a ward manager has no time for "excuses" or possible explanations for poor performance. She expects the best and if she doesn't get it someone will have to pay!

Opportunistic

Opportunistic leaders use a combination of the other Grid styles on the basis of what is likely to help them get ahead. In their dealing with others, they work from the question of what Grid style is likely to help them get what they want from the other person. Opportunistic oriented behaviour is rooted in self-interest. Why do opportunistic leaders act in this way? At one extreme is the desire to be in control and at the other there is a fear of exposure.

Grid Style Consistency and Flexibility

There is a Grid style consistency in that people tend to deal with others in more or less the same way, even over long periods. Despite this relative consistency, there are exceptions in which people may switch temporarily from one style to another before returning to their typical style of relating. The stable mode of relating is referred to as the *dominant* style and the flexibility of shifting to another style is referred to as a *backup* style. The shift to backup style is spontaneous, frequently in situations of crisis, stress, conflict or new environments.

The dominant style is the one most characteristic of people, the one we know and anticipate of them. With the exception of opportunism, each of the six styles is relatively consistent, regardless of the situation or people involved. Some may think that Grid styles do not work when a crisis arises, but most leaders do not pick and choose an approach each time they are faced with a new situation. They respond in an instinctive way to questions, decisions, conflicts and so on. The approach reflects the individual's motivations, past experiences, feelings, values and desires.

In some situations, when a dominant style is not effective a person may shift temporarily to a backup style. For example, mild-mannered 1,9 oriented leaders may suddenly lose their temper and shout at someone. The sudden change probably shocks both parties. The leader will most likely return to the dominant style when the temporary circumstances pass, with an apology and explanation for the unusual behaviour. There are times when managers give up, get annoyed, patronise and so on especially when they do not feel they have the energy to keep listening and helping an individual. While leaders may have clear 9,9 desires about what they want to achieve, their own frailty and lack of skill means that they do not always live that out. A more serious reason may be a lack of self-awareness as to their motivations, hence the motivational scale attached to each behavioural style. Therefore, an important area of learning for leaders is their self-awareness of what their dominant and backup styles are and developing skills in working with others to achieve desired outcomes.

What the Grid teaches us is that leadership requires attention to both task and relational issues and a self-knowledge on the part of leaders as to what motivates their behaviour. Such self-knowledge and skills provide the basis for leader behaviour that is grounded in three areas of competence (Schein, 1978):

1. *Analytical competence*: The ability to identify, analyse and solve problems under conditions of incomplete information and uncertainty
2. *Interpersonal competence*: The ability to influence, supervise and lead people at all levels in the organisation
3. *Emotional competence*: The capacity to be stimulated by emotional and interpersonal issues rather than be debilitated or exhausted by them, the capacity to bear high levels of responsibility without becoming paralysed and the ability to exercise power without guilt

THE LEADER'S ROLE IN CHANGE

In chapter 7 we presented a framework for large system change. This framework outlined five key tasks of moving change through a system, such as an organisation, a team or a unit.

1. Determining the need for change.
2. Defining the desired future state.
3. Assessing the present in terms of the desired future to determine the changes to be made.
4. Implementing the change and managing the transition.
5. Consolidating and sustaining the change.

The task of leadership is to steer the system through the five tasks (Beckhard and Pritchard, 1992). Each task makes its own demands on leadership, which we will now discuss.

Determining the Need for Change

One of the core tasks of any leader is to devote attention to possible changes coming from the external environment. As Hesselbein, Goldsmith and Beckhard (1996) put it, leaders are expected to be constantly "scanning beyond the horizon". Leaders need structures that enable them to determine the need for change. Some of these structures are formal, such as reading research reports, policy documents, consulting experts who are engaged in forecasting and trend analysis, and attending seminars and meetings. Others are informal, such as networking and chatting to other leaders about what they see as emerging.

In terms of what we discussed in chapter 8, an important aspect of a leader's role is to unfreeze the system and to do it in such a manner that the sense of disconfirmation and appropriate anxiety are accompanied by creation of a sense of psychological safety. It is easy for a leader to create disconfirmation and anxiety, and as such to evoke learning anxiety and therefore set the tone for resistance through a 9,1 Grid style. A 9,9 approach that faces the need for change and the dispositions of staff is consistent with good task and people management.

Defining the Desired Future State

The vision of an end state is essentially a statement of leadership's priorities and commitments. There are four aspects to vision-driven change (Beckhard and Pritchard, 1992):

1. Creating and setting the vision.
2. Communicating the vision.
3. Building commitment to the vision.
4. Organising people and what they do so that they are aligned to the vision.

So for leaders, developing a vision and being committed to it, and ensuring the vision is communicated clearly around the organisation are critical. In terms of the systems approach and Burke-Litwin model we discussed in chapter 4, this means creating and leading a sense of common purpose across a system whose parts are in delicate balance with one another. One might imagine that creating this common purpose should be relatively easy in an organisation that exists to provide treatment and care to patients. In reality there are many subgoals within the system that may be in conflict, with each professional group being acutely aware of the need to promote its own profession and way of working, even when this conflicts with another professional group's approach.

Assessing the Present in Terms of the Desired Future to Determine the Changes to be Made

As we saw in earlier chapters, assessment of the present is fraught with political difficulties as the interdepartmental group, teams and individuals may experience this assessment activity as a criticism of their own work and may react defensively and engage in blaming others. Hence the importance of what we explored in chapter 6 – grounding assessments in solid data. Here there is a clear need for 9,9 behaviour so as to avoid the painful conflicts of interests coming from staff (9,1) or being subservient to them in the interests of harmony (1,9) or settling for what one can get away with (5,5).

Implementing the Change and Managing the Transition

As we saw in chapter 7, the transition state is characterised by uncertainty and so leaders need to attend to the dynamics of the transition state through creating enabling structures, building commitment and modelling behaviour. Important questions for executive leaders in this phase of change concern the choices they make about their role. Will they act as project manager of the change or as facilitator? How will they choose which role to play? What messages do they want to communicate by their behaviour? What will they choose to do themselves? What will they manage?

Consolidating and Sustaining the Change

Consolidating and sustaining change is probably the most important task for the leader. Ignoring this aspect of the change process is the most common cause of failure in change initiatives. The pace of change in health services creates its own difficulties for the task of consolidation. New initiatives are implemented in quick succession, leaving little time for consolidation. Buchanan et al. (1999) write about "initiative fatigue" as a concept that has two dimensions:

1. A personal sense of overload and not being able to cope with new demands or consolidate and learn from experiences.
2. Disillusionment and cynicism in the face of forthcoming initiatives.

They term the latter "the BOHICA syndrome (Bend over, here it comes again) – the apathetic response to change which is perceived to be enforced without clear purpose" (1999: 25). They found support for this in the results of a survey which included 96 managers, with 72 per cent agreeing that "People seem to be suffering from information overload" and 67 per cent agreeing that "People in my organisation have seen so much change, not all beneficial to them, that their main response to communication is cynicism." (1999: 25)

One of the key skills the successful leader exhibits is the ability to "stick at it" until improvements result and the change speaks for itself.

Organisational feedback loops are an essential part of this task. If a change process starts to "go off the rails" this will become evident in the feedback. The leader needs to take the decision to make necessary modifications to maintain the credibility and the chances of success of the initiative or to stay the course and risk a rejection of the initiative further down the line. In the face of increasing pressure to stick to deadlines, and possibly the next initiative already lined up for launch, the easier option is to maintain course, although it is clearly the wrong course. The result is that those involved in the change process lose their sense of ownership in the process and become disinterested and the leader finds him/herself alone.

An equally common scenario in healthcare is the tendency of the leader to latch on to each new initiative with enthusiasm and vigour, only to lose interest and move on to the next "new initiative" with the same enthusiasm, leaving his disillusioned followers in his wake.

Review and Learning

The most important process running through the five tasks is learning in action. Managers tend to be results-oriented rather than learning-oriented. Therefore, as learning and change are part of one another, the leadership of change requires learning, both on the part of the leader and the system. The approaches presented in chapter 3, such as action research, clinical inquiry, reflective practice and action learning, among others, provide valuable mechanisms for engaging in cycles of action and reflection, and so facilitate learning in action (Coghlan, 2002). Supporting and rewarding learning is a valuable investment for any organisation undergoing frequent change. Learning from experience, both successes and failures, helps to avoid reinventing the wheel and allows energy to be channelled to sustaining the momentum of change.

Leaders as Heroes

There is a danger that in focusing on the leader of a change process and exploring the influence of leadership style and leadership characteristics, the leader may be viewed as the hero with success attributed primarily to him/her. One of the problems that this view creates is the sense of dependency that can develop in an organisation. Consequently, when a leader leaves, the organisation feels it cannot maintain the momentum of the change process without its leader. Senge (1997) says that in future we will have to surrender the myth of leaders as isolated heroes and replace it with leadership distributed among diverse individuals and teams sharing responsibility for creating an organisation's future. Goodwin (2000) makes the point that leadership research has traditionally focused on the leader-follower relationship and argues that it needs to change its focus from "person-person to person-context". Earlier, Gilmore (1982) highlighted the importance of context by suggesting that because organisations rarely operate as closed systems the impact of the environment has made boundary management skills critical to the successful exercise of leadership, with work on both the internal and external environments enabling the matching of internal strategic choices without external conditions.

CONCLUSIONS

As Burke (2002) argues, the leadership of change matters. Leaders of change work with both task and people issues. They need to be able to maximise both, rather than play one off against the other. This requires both self-knowledge of the motivations underlying leadership styles and skills to enact the 9,9 style. They need to be congruent; they need to practice what they preach. They need to show how their behaviour matches their words and so be able to enlist support and commitment for the change they are leading.

Case 9.1 Leading the Merger

Martin Casey has just been appointed CEO of ICFID (Integrated Care for the Intellectually Disabled). Martin has a strong background in the voluntary sector, having worked as a social worker with a voluntary organisation for twelve years, then progressing to head of clinical services position, CEO of a small voluntary organisation and his most recent position – CEO of a national voluntary organisation providing services to people with autism. His reputation is that of a "solid" manager who "takes no nonsense" and methodically grows and develops any organisation he is involved in. He has had a number of difficulties with staff unions in the past, but his previous Board attributes this to his ability to play "tough". ICFID is a voluntary organisation employing approximately 800 staff. The organisation has resulted from the integration of three religious-owned voluntary organisations that had all been providing similar services in a city of 850,000. The original organisations were located in three different geographical areas, but there was some overlap in the areas they served. There were also some gaps in the service provided by one of the organisations, with the other two providing almost the full range of available services.

The merger of the three organisations had been difficult for a number of reasons, but primarily because of the different value systems

cont/d

of the three organisations. One of the organisations was considered very progressive and had tailored its services to promote client independence where possible. The other two organisations were more traditional and there remained a strong dependency in their client groups. There were also different religious philosophies in the three organisations. The merger was managed by a CEO who had been appointed specifically for the task, which took two years to complete. He was an "outsider", i.e. had no prior association with any of the organisations, and was considered a charismatic and dynamic leader. On the Leadership Grid he would be categorised as a 4,9, i.e. medium concern for task and high concern for people. This style is reflected in ICFID in that it is now considered to be a good employer that has gained a reputation for attracting and retaining good health professionals. However, it is also perceived to be less efficient in terms of resource utilisation and client numbers than the three organisations independently. This is a source of embarrassment for ICFID's Board of Management, as the rationale for the merger was to have a more streamlined and efficient organisation.

Martin has just had his first meeting with the chairman of the Board (a retired chief executive from the telecommunications sector) who made it very clear that his task as CEO is "to turn this organisation around and increase productivity by a minimum of 35% within two years". Martin is acutely aware of the labour shortage in the healthcare sector and feels the organisation is privileged to have good quality health professionals that are loyal to the organisation. He has been given no indication as to why these "quality" professionals are performing so poorly in terms of client numbers.

Questions
1. Do you think Martin Casey was the right choice for the position of CEO of ICFID? Why?
2. If you were in Martin's shoes what targets would you set for the first six months in post?
3. Describe the process you would put in place to realise the board's expectations, indicating the role staff in the organisation would play in this process.

Clinical Inquiry Exercise 9.1

Consider leaders with whom you have worked.

1. Those you consider to be successful leaders
   a) What do you think they did well?
   b) How did they combine outcome and people issues?

2. Those you consider not to be successful leaders.
   a) What do you think they did that was not successful?
   b) What did they do in terms of outcome and people issues?
   c) What were the effects on the outcomes of the work and the impact on the people?

CHAPTER 10

External and Internal
OD Consultants

A significant element in the whole process of organisation development is the role and function of those who are professionals helping organisations manage change, i.e. organisational consultants. Using professional help is frequently a significant element of a change process. Individuals might attend a therapist or a relevant expert as part of attempting to make a change in their lives. What are organisational consultants? Organisational consultants are generally defined as people whose expertise has been contracted by a client. They may be external or internal to the organisation. The "client" is the organisation or person that initiates or commissions the consultation project. The consultation relationship is typically a voluntary one between a professional helper and a help-seeking client, in which the consultant is attempting to help the client solve some problem. The relationship is perceived to be temporary by both parties and the consultant is an outsider to the client's power system. Consultants, i.e. those who come into organisations in a helping role, can fulfil a wide range of roles from technical expert to process facilitator. Effective helping involves helping in such a way that problems are solved.

Models of Consultation

There are different models of consultancy. The most common ones are those that are based on the expertise of the consultant. Two forms of the expert model can be described (Schein, 1999b). The first is called the *medical* or *doctor-patient model*. In this model the client typically presents the situation to the expert who performs a diagnosis and prescribes a remedy, which the client then implements. An example is when a consultant is asked to analyse bed occupancy in a hospital because the hospital management feels they are not utilising their capacity to maximum effect. The consultant does the analysis and suggests the implementation of two discharge times daily that every ward in the hospital adheres to, leading to better coordination of throughput. The second type of expert consultancy is called the *purchase model*. In this model expertise is purchased. The expert comes in and frequently does the job in person. For example, an expert in the development of patient record systems may be invited in to develop a system for a health board. An IT company is contracted to develop and install the system.

Both these models are grounded in the authoritative expertise of the consultant. The authority is based on the relationship between someone with expertise in a particular area and someone who lacks expertise in that area. Power is based on expertise. Such a relationship has its appropriateness and its faults. Its strength lies in having the expertise in areas of content where there is clear lack of knowledge and expertise internally and no desire to invest in having the necessary skills. For example we buy in electronics skills when equipment breaks down. In the doctor-patient model we are expected to follow the prescription of the expert who understands our illness. It has inherent pitfalls in that we are relying on an external diagnosis that may or may not be accurate. We may find ourselves having to return to the "doctor" when the next "illness" surfaces. We may never learn the skills to solve our own problems, instead becoming dependent on the external consultant. This model of consultancy has been the one most in evidence in health systems until recently. The consultancy agency/external consultant arrived in the organisation, met key stakeholders and then went off to diagnose and suggest a remedy that was presented to the organisation in the form of a report. This ended the contract with the consultancy. With the increasing realisation that this infrequently results in any change or improvement, healthcare managers are turning towards other models of consultation.

PROCESS CONSULTATION

There is a third helping model, *process consultation*. Edgar Schein, the creator of process consultation, defines it as "the creation of a relationship with the client that permits the client perceive, understand and act on process events that occur in the client's internal and external environment in order to improve the situation as defined by the client" (1999b: 20). Schein's underlying assumptions are that managers often do not know what is wrong in an organisation and need a special kind of help to understand what their problems actually are. They often do not know what kinds of assistance consultants can give and so need help in knowing what kind to seek. They need help in being able to identify what needs improving and what does not. They may want to solve the problems themselves but they need assistance in deciding what to do. For example, a manager of a voluntary organisation providing services for people with disabilities may know that she needs to change the culture of the organisation in order to move away from a paternalistic model that creates dependency in their clients towards a culture that supports the independence of clients. However, she may not know how or where to begin in order to achieve such a cultural shift. In process consultation, consultants work jointly with managers so that the managers can learn to see the problems for themselves, share in the understanding and be actively involved in creating their own solutions.

On the basis of such assumptions it can be seen that the process consultation model is in direct contrast with traditional consultation models. These models are based on particular areas of consultant expertise that the client consults for advice and/or expert problem solving. Schein makes this comparison as he places the process consultation approach in juxtaposition with the doctor-patient model and the purchase model. Process consultants, in contrast, are experts in building effective helping relationships that are contingent on working jointly with clients so that the clients can solve their own organisational problems. Finally, process consultants pass on their skills to their clients so that, in essence, managers become process consultants in their own organisations. Schein argues that the process consultation approach to helping constitutes authentic organisation development because it is genuinely client-centred and follows the client's needs through the consultation process. This is contrasted with other helping models in which the consultant pre-designs a set of interventions and the client follows the consultant's interventions. In healthcare the issues that need to be worked on are frequently complex and long-standing problems. The prospect of a neat solution, new model or configuration tends to be much more attractive to managers than the notion of slowly and systematically getting to the root of the problem and building a new model internally. It is often easier, therefore, for both the client and the consultant to adopt the "doctor-patient" model. For example, a health board decided to engage external consultants to review the configuration of acute hospitals in their geographical area, knowing that a large part of the problem was created by too many local hospitals necessitating a wide dispersal of resources. The management of that health board thought it much easier to allow the external consultants to adopt the role of "doctor" and design a solution, than it would be to work collaboratively with the internal politics and agendas to build a solution that was acceptable to everyone involved. The result in this kind of scenario can often be a wonderfully insightful document with a neatly packaged model that is accepted by senior management but rejected by everyone else on the grounds that it is unworkable and does not take adequate account of the existing situation.

In process consultation the guiding principle for the consultant is the collaborative working with the client in a manner that enables the client to develop his/her own diagnosis of the situation and the skills to act on it. The relationship is one where the client primarily defines the issues, sets the agenda and has control of the process and, therefore, can experience psychological success, develop skills, grow in trust of others and create effective group relations through this approach. This is contrasted with the approach where the consultant takes the most prominent role, defines the issues, maintains a professional distance through the power of expertise and, in essence, controls the situation. The attributes of the collaborative consultation approach are conceptually closely related to some counselling precepts. Carl Rogers (1990), in describing the characteristics of a helping relationship, invites those in the helping role to face certain questions about their own dispositions. These dispositions relate to the ability to build trust, to allow oneself experience positive feelings towards the other, to be strong enough in oneself to allow freedom to the other, to be able to enter the world of the other and see things as he/she does, to be free from external evaluation and to allow the other person to be "in the process of becoming". Consultants who lack experience may not feel comfortable adopting this role and mistakenly believe that their reputation depends on finding a quick solution and presenting this clearly to the client. Responding to the client's question, "Tell me how to sort out my outpatients clinic?" with "I do not know how to sort out your clinic but I can help you and your staff to find out how" is far more difficult than saying "I'll spend three days in your clinic and then I'll present a solution".

The critical issue is about how to utilise effective help. Hence, whether to draw on the doctor-patient, purchase or process consultation forms of help depends on the issues for which help is required, the dispositions of those seeking help, and in particular, what they are intending by bringing external consultants into the system. Nevis (1987) draws on an interesting analogy from the crime fiction literature. While the image of the consultant as detective has long been present in OD, Nevis elaborates a specific example by contrasting the nineteenth century detective Sherlock Holmes with the TV character Colombo. Sherlock Holmes is a product of nineteenth century rationalism. He works in a rational, analytical and logical mode with a primary focus on deductive reasoning. He holds great intellectual authority over the local police who after all are the professionals in the field and appear incompetent by comparison. Everything Holmes does is planned and he is always in control. In many respects the psychological contract between many clients and consultants mirrors the Holmes model. Clients hope that a superior intelligent being will enter their system, spot all the things they cannot see and authoritatively solve the crimes. In stark contrast, Lt. Columbo is a product of twentieth-century existentialism. He works through close contact with the protagonists in the case. He is constantly present by wandering around, interacting with everyone and appearing to be disorganised and incompetent. It is his very presence, his close contact and repetitive questions that force the villain to make mistakes and ultimately get trapped. Columbo does not get his man by being removed from the scene and deducing conclusions from his study in Baker Street as Sherlock

Holmes does, but by making things happen through being present and asking questions.

Phases of Consultation

The consultation relationship between client and consultant typically has a number of phases. While these phases are described differently in many texts there are some common strands. The initial phases are those where the client contacts the consultant, the relationship is explored and a formal and psychological contract is set. The psychological contract describes the form the consultation is to take: one based on consultant as expert or as process consultant. Then the setting and methods of work are agreed. For the process consultant, this may involve interviewing and observing, and setting up processes whereby members of the organisation may address task and process issues that pertain to how the organisation functions. Each intervention creates its own opportunity for the consultant to help the client understand what is going on and so set up subsequent interventions. The process then is a cycle of intervention and review until the client is satisfied that the problem has been addressed or sufficient progress has been made. Then there is evaluation and disengagement by the consultant.

INTERNAL OD FACILITATORS

While the use of external consultants and facilitators is a common feature of OD in healthcare organisations, there is a growing utilisation of internal consultation and change facilitation resources (Hartley, Benington and Binns, 1997; Coghlan, Mc Auliffe and Pathe, 2002–3).

There are many advantages of using internal OD facilitators (Steele, 1982; Schwartz, 1984; Hunsaker, 1985; Bor and Miller, 1991; Huffington and Bruning, 1994; Berenbaum, 1997; Coghlan and Brannick, 2001): they know the system and speak the language: they understand the norms and; they can identify with the needs and aspirations of the people in the system; they are familiar figures in the organisation; and they can build continuity and follow up their work. At the same time there are some disadvantages. Internal OD facilitators may lack an objective perspective and be hindered by their past affiliations and record. They may not have an adequate power base and may not have independence of movement to be effective, i.e. they become pigeon-holed in their traditional roles by comments such as "what does an occupational therapist know about the problems we have in theatre". Internal OD facilitators may have limited access because they are insiders: for example, "nurses may find themselves confined to working with nurses". It may be difficult for them to redefine ongoing relationships with fellow organisational members: for example, the manager of a social work department may find it difficult to successfully adopt the role of OD facilitator with her own team because they are guarded about expressing their concerns in her presence. Internal consultants may not be seen as "prophets" in their own organisation and may be undervalued, taken for granted and at times scapegoated. They are dependent on this one organisation of which they are members.

Steele (1982) identifies four conceptual themes for internal OD facilitators:

1. *Focus on process*: Internal OD practice is a process rather than a position. Therefore, seeing work projects as finite, with a beginning, middle and end helps build consistency. Some of the phase models that articulate activities of contracting, entry, diagnosing, planning and taking action, reviewing and terminating are useful in framing project work within the organisation.
2. *System dynamics*: System dynamics are the context for action in organisations where everything is affected by everything else as well as being the target for action. We explored this in chapter 4.
3. *Role analysis*: Viewing roles within systems enables OD facilitators to see how problems are caused by role ambiguity, role conflict, and how role analysis concepts help understand influences in systems and helps depersonalise difficulties.
4. *Personal influence methods*: Encouraging people to listen, to question, to take up issues and work them through, to work collaboratively with others.

He also reflects that in relation to the four themes, uncertainty and ambiguity are a normal part of internal OD facilitators' role, which creates useful opportunities as well as limitations. He notes that measurements of the effectiveness of internal consultants are vague and fuzzy and probably contain conflicting views. He notes that on occasion internal OD facilitators need to make choices about actions that are not guided by policies and job descriptions. These choices need to be made consciously. He emphasises the need for diagnosis – collecting information and analysing causes of problems in relation to both organisational task issues and to their own process of working within the system. In Steele's view, most internal OD facilitators do not apply their diagnostic skills to the latter. He cautions against focusing on single events arguing that it is more effective to focus on changing the pattern of events.

Role Ambiguity for the Internal OD Consultant

As with any consultancy relationship, there is high potential for role ambiguity or role conflict (Ramirez and Bartunek, 1989). First, role ambiguity may occur around *what internal OD facilitators do*. So job description, the temporary nature of many of the projects in which internal OD facilitators engage, the loose definition of the role, possible tension within central organisation or corporate services, to name a few, contribute to such ambiguity. A good example is a case where an internal facilitator was asked by the management team to work with a community care team because they were resisting structural changes proposed by management. The facilitator was formerly a therapist working within this community care team. The teams expectation was that as she understood their difficulties she would be able to "fight their case" with management. Management's expectation was that the facilitator had "good insider knowledge and should be able to persuade the team to accept the changes" and so the internal facilitator is caught in the middle.

Second, *how internal OD facilitators work* creates ambiguity and indeed creates the need to justify their existence. For instance, legitimate initiatives that they take are less confining than those of line managers. Their way of working may challenge organisational norms. For example, an internal facilitator may have a direct reporting relationship to the CEO even though in his previous organisational role he was at middle management level. To his peers it appears "he is acting above his station" as they report to senior managers who in turn report to the CEO.

A third source of ambiguity is *how internal OD facilitators are evaluated*. Standards of performance are likely to be fuzzy. Managers may have little basis for evaluating technical and process competence and performance. Indeed it may be argued that to be successful as an OD facilitator one has to be invisible, such that ultimately the manager takes the credit for the success of the project.

Finally, the long-term career prospects of the member of the organisation who is in the internal facilitator role is typically vague and unclear (Coghlan, Mc Auliffe and Pathe, 2002–3). Buchanan et al. (1999), in a survey of UK managers involved in a change forum, found evidence that the role of the change agent is poorly defined and poorly understood in many organisations. Their contributions are poorly recognised, poorly supported and inadequately rewarded in financial or career terms. The consequences for role ambiguity is likely to be stress, anxiety and self-doubt for the individual and an energy drain into constantly clarifying ambiguities of the daily work role. If role ambiguity is minimised then there is considerable benefit for both the individual and the organisation.

Shaping the Role

Steele (1982) argues strongly that internal OD facilitators need to be proactive about shaping their role, rather than allowing others shape it for them or by waiting for things to happen to them. A role is a set of expectations for a person to do a job effectively. Role expectations are never completely explicit, so trying to get complete and full articulation is fruitless. However, when demands do not feel right or unrealistic expectations are being made then some role clarification and renegotiation are required. There is no one "right" internal consulting role any more than there is any one external consulting role. Effective role definition depends on the organisation's needs, the resources of the consultant and the matching of the two. So internal OD facilitators need to negotiate whether an expert, resource or process role is required in any project.

Steele also places five dilemmas before the internal OD facilitator, which in his view are natural positions in any system:

1. *Helping or controlling*: there can be a dilemma between helping a unit or team do what they want to do and trying to get them to do what the boss thinks they should be doing.
2. *Selling or helping*: this dilemma poses questions about the immediate task of working for a group and having an eye on being successful so that there will be future work.
3. *Doing or learning*: there is a tension between being seen to be working productively and doing things that do not look like work, yet are helping the OD facilitator learn, such as reading, sharing experiences, writing up notes.
4. *Sharing the magic or hiding it*: this dilemma focuses on how OD facilitators pass on their skills to clients, which in OD is one of the key criteria for success.
5. *Being safe or taking risks*: this tension between security and risk is based on a) the power differential between the internal OD facilitator and the manager, b) the uncertainty of the outcome, c) personal embarrassment and d) violating peer norms.

In Steele's view there are two approaches to resolving these dilemmas. One is "role synchronisation", by which he means a choice negotiated between internal OD facilitator and manager, which is what also takes place for external consultants. He notes that some internal OD facilitator activities can irritate the management. These can be: the non-synchronisation of time patterns, such as different time systems, long term vs. short-term perspectives and the OD facilitator's need to hold meetings. Internal OD facilitators may assume inappropriate authority: they may take an arrogant stance or be over-deferent; they may be too abstract or they may not get involved enough and stay in their office too much. Of course, management has an equal propensity to irritate the internal OD facilitators, especially through inappropriate expectations, creating poor conditions for the project, such as limiting access or providing inaccurate or too little information. If they do not meet the OD facilitators' expectations around using resources, keeping promises, not putting things off until a crisis develops, they can irritate them. Management can also exploit the OD facilitators by using them in their own power games or by blackmailing them. The creation of structures whereby the internal OD facilitators can regularly meet their superiors and other internal clients, to get feedback, providing a forum to allow for role renegotiation, is important.

Steele's second approach to resolving the dilemmas is the personal development of the OD facilitator whereby issues like role identification and adoption, personal values and risk taking are part of the ongoing agenda of personal and professional development. The vast majority (99 per cent) of managers (members of an organisation development and change forum who were from public and private sector organisations) agreed that the change agent today needs well-developed negotiating, persuading and influencing skills (Buchanan et al. 1999).

Managing Organisational Politics

While an organisation may have a clearly articulated espoused theory of its values, strategies and plans for moving into the future, the project of organisational change is inherently political as it constitutes a movement from existing conditions. Organisation development has the propensity to be counter-cultural in many organisations because it examines everything, stresses listening, emphasises questioning, fosters courage, incites action, abets reflection and endorses democratic participation. Any or all of these characteristics may be threatening to existing organisational norms. OD interventions because of their participative nature, are likely to make differences in values among the various groups or professions much more salient than they would otherwise be. As a result they are likely to increase the likelihood of conflicts and political behaviours, and cause some people to "win" and others to "lose" (Ramirez and Bartunek, 1989). Many OD interventions are political acts, e.g. giving feedback. Managers and organisational leaders are constantly engaging in political balancing acts in order to achieve their goals. Similarly, internal OD facilitators are engaging in organisational politics, without the benefit of having managerial authority. Change heightens the prevalence and intensity of political action. Many writers argue that change agents should not become involved in organisational politics (Ward, 1994; French and Bell, 1999). Only very few have argued that the change agent should have the skills and expertise to handle political issues (Buchanan and Boddy, 1992; Hardy 1996.)

Cooklin (1999) refers to the insider change agent as the "irreverent inmate" who is a supporter of the people in the organisation, a saboteur of the organisation's rituals and a questioner of some of its beliefs. While internal OD facilitators may see themselves as attempting to generate valid and useful information in order to facilitate free and informed choice so that there will be commitment to those choices in accordance with the theory and practice of organisation development and organisational learning, (Argyris, 1970; Argyris and Schon, 1996), they typically find that, as Kakabadse (1984) argues, what constitutes valid information is intensely political. In a similar vein, Golembiewski (1990) discourages viewing OD as narrowly facilitative as it limits OD facilitators both personally and professionally. He argues that native cunning discourages a view of OD as facilitative as there is a need to avoid a view that OD facilitators are naïve, patsies or Judas goats.

Accordingly, internal OD facilitators need to be politically astute, becoming what Buchanan and Badham (1999) call a "political entrepreneur". In their view, this role implies a behaviour repertoire of political strategies and tactics and a reflective self-critical perspective on how those political behaviours may be deployed. Buchanan and Boddy (1992) describe the management of the political role in terms of two activities, performing and backstaging. *Performing* involves the public performance role of being active in the change process, building participation for change, pursuing the change agenda rationally and logically, while backstage activity involves the recruitment and maintenance of support and the reduction of resistance. *Backstaging* comprises skills at intervening in the political and cultural systems, through justifying, influencing and negotiating, defeating opposition and so on. Internal OD facilitators need to be prepared to work the organisation's political system, by maintaining their credibility as an effective driver of change and as an astute political player. The key to this is assessing the power and interests of relevant stakeholders in relation to aspects of any project. A general manager of a community care area may have a great deal of influence with regard to budget allocation, but little influence with regard to strategic decision making. Another general manager may be adept at instilling loyalty and commitment in colleagues and staff, in contrast to yet another who may be distrusted by everyone. Clearly the choice of which general manager to engage in communicating changes proposed to the community care service is a crucial one in the change process. Several models of change cite "commitment from top management" as a key component, implying that if this is present, the whole organisation will row in behind the change. The politically astute change agent realises this is not the case and works to build commitment. Harrison (1995) suggests working with the forces in the organisation that are supportive of change rather than working against those who are defensive and resistant.

Kakabadse (1984) presents six useful guidelines:

1. *Identify the stakeholders*: identifying those who have a stake or interest in the project and its outcomes and approaching them so as to identify their intentions.
2. *Work on the comfort zones*: working on those behaviours, values and

ideas that a person can accept, tolerate or manage. As long as these are not threatened, people will be able to focus on wider concerns.

3. *Network*: going beyond formal hierarchies or structures, where necessary, to coalitions of interests that may exert greater influence on key stakeholders than the hierarchical structure.

4. *Make deals*: making deals are common in organisations as individuals and groups agree to support one another on a particular issue in return for support on others. This is a common way of reaching agreement on policies.

5. *Withhold and withdraw*: it may be useful on occasion to withhold information in order not to fuel opposition, though withholding information constantly would not be a good thing. It is also useful on occasion to withdraw from conflictual situations and let others sort out the issue.

6. If all else fails, Kakabadse recommends that OD facilitators need to have some *fall-back strategies*.

In order to be able to manage the content and control agendas of the OD project and the power-political processes of influencing and ensuring the legitimacy of their OD work, internal OD facilitators need to be able to manage key stakeholders (Greiner and Schein, 1988; Harrison, 1995; Coghlan and Brannick, 2001). A list of such stakeholders would typically include: the OD facilitator's manager, that manager's own manager, other senior managers and directors, those who are the direct target of the change, their leaders, both formal and informal and so on.

Beckhard and Harris (1987) propose a technique that is useful for mapping significant political relationships with regard to a change project. They have developed a "commitment map" on which key players in the change process are categorised as showing "no commitment", "let it happen" (i.e. the change project), "help it happen" and "make it happen". They suggest that not every player needs to be in the "make it happen" category, but it is useful to decide in which category one would like to have each player and the OD facilitator can then work towards achieving that. The "bacon and eggs" analogy is a good one here – the chicken is clearly involved but the pig is committed!

Internal OD facilitators may pose a number of questions to themselves as they plan where to make their interventions. These questions help create awareness of the systemic nature of the organisation and how interventions may be grounded in the dynamics of the system (Harrison, 1995).

- *Accessibility*: Who is accessible?
- *Leverage*: How much leverage do I have? Will I be able to influence this person?
- *Vulnerability*: Is this person open to change?

- *Appropriateness*: Is it appropriate to work with/through this person, given the structure of the system?
- *Linkage*: What is the target person's linkage to the rest of the system?

ETHICS IN ORGANISATION DEVELOPMENT

Organisation development is a value-driven approach to change management and so it is important that OD facilitators exemplify OD values in their professional behaviour with the people in the systems with which they work (Lippitt and Lippitt, 1978; White and Wooten, 1986; Church, 2001). The work of any professional helper requires the constant exercise of sensitivity, discretion and judgement. OD facilitators work with the vulnerabilities of systems as they confront the challenges, difficulties and pains of change. Accordingly, OD facilitators frequently find themselves in positions in which they have to make choices based on value judgements.

Rothwell et al. (1995) suggest three ways of becoming ethically aware and developing ethical competencies:

1. Knowledge of codes of ethics of organisations concerned with OD, such as OD Network (US), OD Institute, ASTD Code of Ethics (Rothwell et al. reproduce these codes in appendices).
2. Continuing personal reflection and self-awareness, including clarifying one's values and developing ethical relational principles.
3. Conversations with other OD facilitators.

Gellerman, Frankel and Ladenson (1990) articulate four ethical principles for OD:

1. Serve the good of the whole.
2. Treat others as we would like them to treat us.
3. Always treat people as ends, never only as means; respect their being and never use them for their ability to do; treat people as individuals and never as subjects.
4. Act so we do not increase power by more powerful stakeholders over less powerful.

One of the main sources of ethical dilemmas for OD facilitators is through what White and Wooten (1986) refer to as "role episode" by which they mean studying an ethical dilemma through an ambiguity or conflict between the sending role and role receiver. The *sending role* comprises expectations of what the OD facilitator role will fulfil. The *receiving role* has perceptions of both the role and of the sending role and then either complies or resists. White and Wooten apply the role episode model to five categories of ethical dilemmas: misrepresentation and collusion, misuse of data, manipulation and coercion, values and goals conflict, and technical ineptness. Also Bate (2000a: 488), in describing the role of an external consultancy team working on culture change in a large hospital, highlights the importance of neutrality and even-handedness.

> We were positioned in the space between management and workforce, strenuously avoiding being seen as either management-centric or worker-centric, acting as knowledge workers...and mediating between the different interests and perspectives to facilitate the development and implementation of collaborative strategies for change.

OD facilitators face a fundamental dilemma: manipulating human behaviour violates a fundamental value yet effective behavioural change requires the use of power and influence in exerting influence on others (Lippitt and Lippitt, 1978). While the base of that power is not coercive or legitimate but rather expert and facilitative, it is nonetheless real and OD facilitators need to be aware of it and address it for themselves (Greiner and Schein, 1988).

Generally speaking ethical guidelines for external and internal OD facilitators are much the same. Any critical difference lies in internal OD facilitators being aware of and confronting their prior experience of the organisation, responsibilities, loyalties, and fears about their future career. In the healthcare sector the ethical dilemmas may be further complicated by the need to continually assess the potential impact of any change in the welfare of patients or clients. At the most basic level this may involve a cost benefit analysis of time out from patient care now working on a strategy to improve patient care in the future.

Case 10.1 Ethical Dilemma

An OD facilitator is meeting with the manager of a health unit where staff are demoralised by impending budget cuts. The board, at its last meeting, expressed displeasure at evidence of staff discontent and the way the manager is handling the situation. The manager says, "Off the record, I need to tell you something that's going on with the board chairman and some of his cronies that's really aggravating the mess I'm in."

Role dilemma for OD facilitator: Should she accept the "off the record" contract or intervene at this moment to refuse this kind of commitment?

cont/d

Decision-Action Alternatives

1. Accept the request for confidentiality.
2. Interpret the contract with the total client system as requiring that she uses her discretion on what is the best use of all the data she receives.
3. Agree to the confidence but indicate she may want to get his voluntary release for her to use it if she sees the value of this and if he agrees.
4. Others she might see?

Value Criteria

1. Not to get trapped into having important data and not being free to use it.
2. Not supporting norms of secrecy that inhibit development of open communication between the parts of the system.
3. Need to be a trusted recipient of controversial data in order to contribute to adequate diagnosis.
4. Others she might consider?

Decisions and Actions of OD Facilitator

- Ask him if he would refrain from prejudging the best use of his opinions, feelings and observations, that she was not committed to doing anything that would be harmful to his relations with the board and staff and so would recommend what she saw might be helpful.
- After hearing his observations and belief about a clique in the board attempting to go behind his back and conspiring to oust him, she suggests she would like to talk to board members and staff to get their assessment of the situation, indicating that she had already talked to him with the idea of convening a problem-sharing meeting to give feedback on her perception of the problems to be faced.

Some Value Principles

- The invoking of the "confidentiality ethic" is usually motivated by the felt need for self-protection or distrust of others to make professional use of the data. This is usually dysfunctional to good problem solving and OD process.
- To be loaded with the commitment of confidentiality may put one in the undesirable role of being a poor substitute for open communication.

cont/d

- To be perceived as a repository for confidential information can be interpreted as being the role of advocacy or being on one side leading to loss of credibility as an objective helper.

Some Skills Utilised

- The skill of inhibiting the natural personal inclination to respond positively to the offer of confidential sharing.
- The skill of helping the client see and accept the wider perspective of the whole system and the OD facilitator's facilitative role.
- The skill of communicating the value of conflict management approaches and constructive communication.

Hunsaker (1985) provides ten principles of being a successful insider change agent:

1. Know yourself.
2. Understand the organisation.
3. Keep lines of communication open.
4. Determine how others feel.
5. Analyse situations from as many points of view as you can.
6. Have a thorough understanding of all the dimensions of a proposed change.
7. Be persistent and continually try to make inroads whenever opportunities present themselves.
8. Develop a sense of timing.
9. Share credit with others.
10. Avoid win-lose strategies.

Friedman (2001) suggests four attributes: be proactive and reflective; be critical and committed; be independent and work well with others and have aspirations; and be realistic about limits. In policy terms, Harrison (1995) suggests working in pairs or teams so that an internal facilitator does not have to work alone in high-risk or high-stress situations. He also argues for building personal and professional support systems among internal OD facilitators.

Shepard (1997) provides a few rules of thumb for change agents:

- *Stay alive*: care for yourself. Keep a life outside of the project and so maintain the ability to turn yourself on and off. Stay in touch with the purpose of the project and go with the flow.
- *Start where the system is*: have empathy with the system and the people in it, particularly as it will not like being "diagnosed".
- *Never work uphill*: keep working at collaboration and work in the most promising arena.

- *Innovation requires a good idea, initiative and a few friends*: find the people who are ready to work on the project and get them working together.
- *Load experiments with success*: work at building success steps along the way.
- *Light many fires*: remember the notion of systems. Any part of a system is the way it is because of how the rest of the system is. As you work towards change in one part, other parts will push the system back to the way it was. Understand the interdependencies among subsystems and keep movement going in as many of them as you can.
- *Keep an optimistic bias*: stay focused on vision and desired outcomes.
- *Capture the moment*: stay in tune with yourself and the situation.

Conclusions

All organisations need help with change at some time or other. On some occasions they may need expert help to offer advice or to conduct training. On other occasions it may need outside facilitator help, i.e. the kind of help that enables managers to do their own organisational diagnosis, make their own change plans and think things through. On occasion the organisation benefits from having these skills in-house. What is important is that whatever help an organisation receives, be it expert or facilitative, external or internal, this help is effective at enabling the organisation make changes as it sees fit and develop its capability to manage change continuously as required by today's world.

Case 10.2 Relationship between Board and Executive at St Fintan's Hospital

The chairman of the Board of St. Fintan's hospital, Michael Catrell telephoned an external consultant, Mary Sullivan (who had been recommended to him by a colleague of his), and asked if she could help the board and executive team to work better together. Mary met Michael to discuss the project in order to establish if she could provide assistance. Michael explained that he had become chairman of the hospital board six months previously and, because it was all so new to him, it had taken him until now to realise that the tensions that exist between the board and the executive management of the hospital are creating difficulties in terms of the prioritisation of problems to be dealt with and the effective management of the hospital. He also feels that the executive management team and the board do not have a shared vision. He elaborated on this by explaining that the board has ideas for developing and expanding the hospital, but these are not being taken up

contl/d

by the executive because they are too busy managing the day-to-day crises. He did suggest to Jim Robbins, the CEO, about two months ago that the board and executive should have a planning weekend, but Jim's reply was that they could not afford it and anyhow he did not think they needed it as they had their service plans submitted for the forthcoming year and these had been approved by the board.

Michael explained the reason he was asking for help now and assured her he was doing this with Jim's agreement. At the last Board meeting, the director of planning, Liam Gallagher, who is on the executive, presented plans for the new wing of the hospital to the board. Dr Carmel Finlay, a GP on the board, interrupted his presentation to point out that the proposed external façade of the building appeared "cold and unwelcoming and isn't in keeping with the image the hospital should be portraying". Liam's response was "with all due respect I think the façade is an issue for the architects and they seem to know what they are doing". Carmel let this pass, but after the meeting she came to Michael to complain about Liam suggesting that maybe he wasn't competent to fulfil the role of director of planning if he didn't think it appropriate to challenge the architect. Michael relayed this conversation to Jim who agreed that a team-building day for the board and executive might be a good idea.

Mary agreed to take on the task but said she would like to meet Jim and would then work on a design or plan for the team-building day. She established that the executive consisted of CEO, deputy CEO, director of finance, director of planning, chair of medical board, director of nursing, director of information systems and director of human resource management. The board consisted of the executive plus a GP, a medical consultant and a nurse (employed by the hospital), two politicians, a local teacher, a retired businessman and the chairman (also retired from the IT sector).

Mary found Jim to be a very likeable personality who seemed genuinely committed to improving the hospital. He seemed to have a lot of respect for his executive team. He acknowledged that they had some difficulties with the Board, but these had only arisen after Michael had taken over as chairman. He hinted that Michael was interfering too much in the operational running of the hospital, adding that there was something she probably did not know about Michael. He then paused before assuring her that he didn't want to be telling tales out of school. The information that Jim was about to provide was that Michael had recently started an affair with the director of nursing.

Questions
1. As an external consultant (i.e. Mary) design a process and team-building day to diagnose the problems in the team and help them build a better working relationship?
2. Would you approach this any differently if you were an internal

cont/d

consultant in the organisation who was not part of the executive?
3. Considering the issues we have discussed in this chapter relating to role and ethics of consultancy, how would you handle the scenario where the CEO is offering information about the chairman?

Clinical Inquiry Exercise 10.1

Reflect on a situation with which you are familiar in which external consultant(s) were used.

- Why were they brought in?
- What were they asked to do?
- Under what model of consultation were they asked to work? Was this what was expected and wanted in the organisation?
- What did they do during the consultation period?
- What was the reaction to their presence and work?
- What were the outcomes, both intended and unintended?
- What were the long-term outcomes of the consultation?
- What have you learned from having external consultants that you would want a) to repeat in the future and b) avoid in the future?

Clinical Inquiry Exercise 10.2

Repeat Clinical Exercise 10.1 for a situation in which an internal OD facilitator was used.

A Final Word

We have approached the subject of change management in healthcare systems through the framework of organisation development. The value base that underlies OD, an approach to working change through a system that is grounded in respecting the individual and helping teams and groups work, makes it particularly appropriate for changing healthcare organisations who depend heavily on teamwork and the engagement and cooperation of the various healthcare professionals. The emphasis on people in systems that OD is built upon complements the values espoused by the health system. Individual professionals in the healthcare system have all been subjected to change of one kind or another, and will continuously be expected to embrace change in the future. The "initiative fatigue" we referred to in chapter 9 is a major problem for healthcare organisations today. This fatigue is exacerbated by the persistent pattern of failed change efforts. Healthcare professionals become disaffected when they are not actively engaged in the planning and initiation of change efforts and when they inevitably are expected to take the blame for failed change initiatives. OD, as an approach to change management, distinguishes itself from other approaches because it requires the involvement from the outset of all those making the change. It thus reduces the risk of disaffection and fatigue.

Within OD action research is paramount. At its core action research begins with experience and works back to understanding and theory development through engagement in cycles of reflection and action. This cyclical process is key to both individual and organisational learning. Learning is critical to success in change efforts. Too often the pain of failure prevents any retrospective learning after the change initiative has been (usually unsuccessfully) completed. The action research component of OD ensures that learning is an inbuilt part of the change process. Accordingly, we have framed our approach by inviting readers to engage in reflection-in-action in order that they might learn-in-action, rather than simply engage with the concepts in this book in a notional way. This is a discipline that healthcare professionals and particularly those who manage health services would do well to develop.

We hope this book will encourage healthcare organisations and the individuals within them to rethink how they approach change, and in doing so create space for learning and developing internal capacity. Much work remains to be done in the health system as to how change can be introduced, implemented and sustained, and how organisation development expertise can be utilised in this work. We hope this book, through its integration of theory and practice, will serve to develop the dialogue between researchers, policy makers and healthcare professionals that is necessary for further advancement of knowledge in the critical area of changing healthcare organisations.

References

Adair, J. (1990) *Not Bosses but Leaders*. Kogan Page: London.

Ancona, D. and Caldwell, D. (1988) "Beyond Task and Maintenance: Defining External Functions in Groups." *Group and Organisation Studies*, 13 (4), 468–94.

Anderson, V. and Johnson, L. (1997) *Systems Thinking Basics: From Concepts to Causal Loops*. Pegasus: Cambridge, MA.

Argyris, C. (1960) *Understanding Organisational Behavior*. Tavistock: London.

Argyris, C. (1970) *Intervention Theory and Method*. Addison-Wesley: Reading, MA.

Argyris, C. (1985) *Strategy, Change and Defensive Routines*. Pitman: Marshfield, MA.

Argyris, C. (1990a) *Integrating the Individual and the Organisation*. With a new introduction by the author. Transaction: New Brunswick, NJ.

Argyris, C. (1990b) *Overcoming Organisational Defenses*. Allyn and Bacon: Boston.

Argyris, C. and Schon, D. (1996) *Organisational Learning II*. Addison-Wesley: Reading, MA.

Argyris, C., Putnam, R. and Smith, D. (1985) *Action Science*. Jossey-Bass: San Francisco.

Armstrong, M. (1999) "Leadership and Mentoring in the Irish Health Services: An Exploration of Gender Differences." Unpublished M.Sc. Thesis. University of Dublin: Dublin.

Ashforth, B. and Lee R. (1990) "Defensive Behavior in Organisations: A Preliminary Model." *Human Relations*, 43 (7), 621–48.

Barker, S.B. and Barker, R.T. (1994) "Managing Change in an Interdisciplinary Inpatient Unit, An Action Research Approach." *Journal of Mental Health Administration*, 21 (1), 80–91.

Bass, B.M. and Avolia, B.J. (1994) (eds) *Leadership Theory and Research Perspectives and Directions*. Academic Press: NewYork.

Bate, P. (2000a) "Changing the Culture of a Hospital: From Hierarchy to Networked Community." *Public Administration*, 78 (3), 485–512.

Bate, P. (2000b) "Synthesizing Research and Practice: Using the Action Research Approach in Health Care Settings." *Social Policy and Administration*, 34 (4), 478–93.

Beckhard, R. (1969) *Organisation Development: Strategies and Models*. Addison-Wesley: Reading, MA.

Beckhard, R. (1997a) "The Healthy Organisation" in F. Hesselbein, M.

Goldsmith and R. Beckhard (eds) *The Organisation of the Future.* Jossey-Bass: San Francisco, 325–28.

Beckhard, R. (1997b) *Agent of Change, My Life, My Work.* Jossey-Bass: San Francisco.

Beckhard, R. and Harris, R. (1987) *Organisational Transitions: Managing Complex Change.* (1st ed. 1977) Addison-Wesley: Reading, MA.

Beckhard, R. and Pritchard, W. (1992) *Changing the Essence: The Art of Creating and Leading Fundamental Change in Organisations.* Jossey-Bass: San Francisco.

Beer, M., Eisenstat, R. and Spector, B. (1990) "Why Change Programs Don't Produce Change." *Harvard Business Review,* November–December, 158–66.

Belbin, R.M. (1981) *Management Teams: Why They Succeed or Fail.* Heinemann: London.

Bennis, W.G. (1969) *Organisation Development: Its Nature, Origins and Prospects.* Addison-Wesley: Reading, MA.

Berenbaum, R. (1997) "Internal Consultancy" in J. Neumann, K. Kellner and A. Dawson-Shepherd (eds) *Developing Organisational Consultancy.* Routledge: London, 71–89.

Blake, R. and McCanse, A. (1991) *Leadership Dilemmas – Grid Solutions.* Gulf: Houston, Tx.

Blake, R. and Mouton, J. (1964) *The Managerial Grid.* Gulf: Houston, Tx.

Blake, R. and Mouton, J. (1978) *The New Managerial Grid.* Gulf: Houston, Tx.

Blake, R., Mouton, J. and Tapper, M. (1981) *Grid Approaches for Managerial Leadership in Nursing.* Mosby: St Louis.

Bolman, D. and Deal, T. (1999) *Reframing Organisations,* 2nd ed. Jossey-Bass: San Francisco.

Bor, R. and Miller, R. (1991) *Internal Consultation in Health Care Settings.* Karnac: London.

Boss, W.R. (1989) *Organisation Development in Health Care.* Addison-Wesley: Reading, MA.

Bowling, A. (2000) *Research Methods in Health: Investigating Health and Health Services.* Buckingham: Open University Press.

Brown, L.D. and Covey, J.G (1987) "Development Organisations and Organisation Development" in R.W. Woodman and W.A. Pasmore (eds) *Research in Organisational Change and Development,* Vol. 1, JAI: Greenwich, CT, 59–88.

Buchanan, D. (1997) "The Limitations and Opportunities of Business Process Re-engineering in a Politicized Organisational Climate." *Human Relations,* 50 (1), 51–72.

Buchanan, D. and Badham, R. (1999) *Power, Politics and Organisational Change.* Sage: London.

Buchanan, D. and Boddy, D. (1992) *The Expertise of the Change Agent.* Prentice-Hall: London.

Buchanan, D., Claydon, T. and Doyle, M. (1999) "Organisation Development and Change: The Legacy of the Nineties." *Human Resource Management Journal*, 9 (2), 20–37.

Bunker, B.B. and Alban, B. (1997) *Large Group Interventions.* Jossey-Bass: San Francisco.

Burke, W.W. (1994) *Organisation Development: A Process of Learning and Changing.* Addison-Wesley: Reading, MA.

Burke, W.W. (2002) *Organisation Change: Theory and Practice.* Sage: Thousand Oaks, CA.

Burke, W.W. and Litwin, G.H. (1992) "A Causal Model of Organisational Performance and Change." *Journal of Management*, 18 (3), 532–45.

Burns, J.M. (1978) *Leadership.* Harper and Row: New York.

Burns, T. and Stalker, G. (1961) *The Management of Innovation.* Tavistock: London.

Bushe, G. and Shani, A.R (1991) *Parallel Learning Structures: Increasing Innovation in Bureaucracies.* Addison-Wesley: Reading, MA.

Cameron, K. (1980) "Critical Questions in Assessing Organisational Effectiveness." *Organisational Dynamics*, 9 (2), 66–80.

Campbell, D., Coldicott, T. and Kinsella, K. (1994) *Systemic Work with Organisations: A New Model for Managers and Change Agents.* Karnac: London.

Campbell, D., Draper, R. and Huffington, C. (1991) *A Systemic Approach to Consultation.* Karnac: London.

Carney, M. (1999) "Leadership in Nursing: Where Do We Go from Here? The Ward Sister's Challenge for the Future." *Nursing Review*, 17 (1–2), 18–24.

Cartwright, D. (1989) "Achieving Change in People: Some Applications of Group Dynamics Theory" in W. French, C. Bell and R. Zawacki (eds) *Organisation Development: Theory, Practice and Research*, 3rd ed. BPI-Irwin: Homewood, IL, 113–21.

Chin, R. and Benne, K. (1985) "Strategies for Effecting Planned Change in Human Systems" in W. Bennis, K. Benne and R. Chin, *The Planning of Change*, 4th ed. Holt, Rinehart and Winston: New York, 22–45.

Chow, C.W., Ganulin, D., Teknika, O., Haddad, K. and Williamson, J. (1998) "The Balanced Scorecard: A Potent Tool for Energizing and Focusing Healthcare Organisation Management." *Journal of Healthcare Management*, 43 (3), 263–80.

Church, A.C. (2001) "The Professionalization of Organisation Development: The Next Step in an Evolving Field" in R. Woodman and W. Pasmore (eds) *Research in Organisational Change and Development*, Vol. 13, JAI: Greenwich, CT, 1–42.

Church, A.C. and Waclawski, J. (2001) *Designing and Using Organisational Surveys: A Seven-Step Process.* Jossey-Bass: San Francisco.

Coghlan, D. (1997) "Organisational Learning as a Dynamic Inter-Level Process" in M.A. Rahim, R.T. Golembiewski and L.E. Pate (eds) *Current Topics in Management*, Vol. 2, JAI Press: Greenwich, CT, 27–44.

Coghlan, D. (1998) "The Process of Change through Interlevel Dynamics in a Large-Group Intervention for a Religious Organisation." *Journal of Applied Behavioural Science*, 34 (1), 105–19.

Coghlan, D. (2000a) "The Interlevel Dynamics of Large System Change." *Organisation Development Journal*, 18 (1), 41–50.

Coghlan, D. (2000b) "Perceiving, Evaluating and Responding to Change: An Interlevel Approach" in R.T Golembiewski (ed.) *Handbook of Organisational Consultation*, 2nd ed. Marcel Dekker: New York, 213–17.

Coghlan, D. (2002) "Developing Organisations through Reflective Practice in Healthcare Systems." *Journal of Irish Colleges of Physicians and Surgeons*, 31 (4), 238–42.

Coghlan, D. and Brannick, T. (2001) *Doing Action Research in Your Own Organisation.* Sage: London.

Coghlan, D. and Casey, M. (2001) "Research from the Inside: Challenges of Doing Action Research in Your Own Hospital." *Journal of Advanced Nursing*, 35, 674–82

Coghlan, D. and Rashford, N.S. (1990) "Uncovering and Dealing with Organisational Distortions." *Journal of Managerial Psychology*, 5 (3), 17–21.

Coghlan, D., Mc Auliffe, E. and Pathe, A. (2002–3) "Internal Organisation Development and Change Practitioners in the Irish Health Boards. Current Practices and Issues." *Administration*, 51 (4), 81–101.

Cooklin, A. (1999) *Changing Organisations: Clinicians as Agents of Change.* Karnac: London.

Cooper, J. and Hewison, A. (2002) "Implementing Audit in Palliative Care: An Action Research Approach." *Journal of Advanced Nursing*, 39, 360–69.

Cooperrider, D., Sorensen, P., Whitney, D. and Yaeger, T. (2000) *Appreciative Inquiry: Rethinking Human Organisation toward a Positive Theory of Change.* Stipes: Champaign, IL.

Cummings, T. and Worley, C. (2001) *Essentials of Organisation Development and Change.* South-Western: Cincinnati.

Cunningham, J.B. (1993) *Action Research and Organisation Development.* Praeger: New York.

Cutliffe, J.R and Basser, C. (1997) "Introducing Change in Nursing: The

Case of Research." *Journal of Nursing Management*, 5, 241–47.

D'Art, D. and Turner, T. (2002) *Irish Employment Relations in the New Economy*. Blackhall: Dublin.

Dannemiller and Associates (2000) *Real Time Strategic Change*. Berrett-Kohler: San Francisco.

Department of Health and Children (2001) *Quality and Fairness: A Health Strategy for You*. Stationary Office: Dublin.

DiBella, A.J. (2001) *Learning Practices*. Prentice-Hall: Upper Saddle River, NJ.

Dixon, M. and Baker, A. (1996) *A Management Development Strategy for the Health and Personal Social Services in Ireland*. Department of Health and Children: Dublin.

Dixon, N. (1994) *The Organisational Learning Cycle*. McGraw-Hill: Maidenhead.

Dunphy, D. and Stace, D. (1990) "Transformational and Coercive Strategies for Planned Organisational Change: Beyond the OD Model" in F. Massarik (ed.) *Advances in Organisation Development*, Vol. 1 Ablex: Norwood, NJ, 85–104.

Emery, F. and Purser, R. (1996) *The Search Conference*. Jossey-Bass: San Francisco.

Farias, G. and Johnson, H. (2000) "Organisation Development and Change Management: Setting the Record Straight." *Journal of Applied Behavioral Science*, 36 (3), 376–81.

Fedoruk, M. and Pincombe, J. (2000) "The Nurse Executive: Challenges for the 21st Century." *Journal of Nursing Management*, 8, 13–20.

Ferlie, E. (1997) "Large Scale Organisational and Management Change in Healthcare: A Review of the Literature." *Journal of Health Services Research and Policy*, 2 (3), 180–89.

Fisher, R. and Ury, W. (1986) *Getting to Yes*. Business Books: London.

Flanagan, J. (1954) "The Critical Incident Technique." *Psychology Bulletin*, 51, 327–58.

Flint, H. (2001) "Nursing Development Units: Progress and Developments." *Nursing Standard*, 15 (29) 39–41.

Fox, A. (1985) *Man Mismanagement*. Hutchinson: London.

Freeman, C. and Penrod, P. (1993) "Applying OD and TQM Strategies to Manage Change in Hospitals." *Organisation Development Journal*, 11 (4), 61–9.

French, W. and Bell, C. (1999) *Organisation Development*, 6th ed. Prentice-Hall: Upper Saddle River, NJ.

Friedman, V. (2001) "The Individual as Agent of Organisational Learning" in M. Dierkes, J. Child, I. Nonaka and A. Berthoin (eds) *Handbook of Organisational Learning*. Oxford University Press: Oxford, 398–414.

Gellerman, W., Frankel, M. and Ladenson, R. (1990) *Values and Ethics in Organisation Development and Human Systems Development: Responding to Dilemmas in Professional Life.* Jossey-Bass: San Francisco.

Gibbon, B. and Little, V. (1995) "Improving Stroke Care through Action Research." *Journal of Clinical Nursing*, 4, 93–100.

Gilmore, T.N. (1982) "Leadership and Boundary Management." *Journal of Applied Behavioral Science*, 18 (3), 342–56.

Goldstein, J. (1989) "The Affirmative Core of Resistance." *Organisation Development Journal*, 7 (1), 32–8.

Golembiewski, R.T. (1989) *Organisation Development: Ideas and Issues.* Transaction: New Brunswick.

Golembiewski, R.T. (1990) "OD as Facilitative and Political." *Organisation Development Journal*, 8 (2), 6–9.

Goodwin, N. (2000) "Leadership and the UK Health Service." *Health Policy*, 51, 49–60.

Greenwood, D. and Levin, M. (1998) *Introduction to Action Research.* Sage: Thousand Oaks, CA.

Greiner, L. and Schein, V.E. (1988) *Power and Organisation Development.* Addison-Wesley: Reading, MA.

Gunnigle, P., McMahon, G. and Fitzgerald G. (1999) *Industrial Relations in Ireland: Theory and Practice.* Gill and Macmillan: Dublin.

Haffer, A. (1986) "Facilitating Change: Choosing the Appropriate Strategy." *Journal of Nursing Administration*, 16 (4), 6–10.

Hamblin, B., Keep, J. and Ash K. (2001) *Organisational Change and Development.* Pearson: London.

Hanson, P. and Lubin, B. (1995) *Answers to Questions Most Frequently Asked about Organisation Development.* Sage: Thousands Oaks, CA.

Hardy, C. (1996) "Understanding Power: Bringing About Strategic Change." *British Journal of Management*, 7, 3–16.

Harrison, M. (1994) *Diagnosing Organisations*, 2nd ed. Sage: Thousand Oaks, CA.

Harrison, M. and Shirom, A. (1999) *Organisational Diagnosis and Assessment.* Sage: Thousand Oaks, CA.

Harrison, R. (1995) "Strategy Guidelines for an Internal Organisation Development Unit" in *The Collected Papers of Roger Harrison.* Jossey-Bass: San Francisco, 33–41.

Harrison, R.G. and Robertson, M. (1985) "Organisation Development: An Alternative Strategy for Organisational Renewal in the NHS?" *Hospital and Health Services Review*, May, 125–29.

Hart, E. and Bond, M. (1995) *Action Research for Health and Social Care: A Guide to Practice.* Open University Press: Milton Keynes.

Hartley, J., Benington, J. and Binns, P. (1997) "Researching the Roles of Internal-change Agents in the Management of Organisational

Change." *British Journal of Management*, 8, 61–73.

Health Services Partnership Agreement (2000) Health Services Partnership Forum, www.healthservicepf.ie

Heron, J. (1996) *Cooperative Inquiry*. Sage: London.

Heslop, L., Elsom, S. and Parker, N. (2000) "Improving Continuity of Patient Care Across Psychiatric Emergency Services: Combing Patient Data with a Participatory Action Research Framework." *Journal of Advanced Nursing*, 31, 135–43.

Hesselbein, F., Goldsmith, M. and Beckhard, R. (1996) *The Leader of the Future*. Jossey-Bass: San Francisco.

Holter, I. and Schwartz-Barcott, D. (1993) "Action Research: What It Is and How It Can be Used in Nursing." *Journal of Advanced Nursing*, 18, 298–304.

Howard, A. and Associates (1994) *Diagnosis for Organisational Change*. Guildford: New York.

Huffington, C. and Bruning, H. (1994) *Internal Consultancy in the Public Sector*. Karnac: London.

Hunsaker, P. (1985) "Strategies for Organisational Change: Role of the Inside Change Agent" in D.D. Warrick (ed.) *Contemporary Organisation Development*. Scott Foresman: Glenview, IL, 123–37.

Hussey, D.E. (1995) *How to Manage Change*. Kogan Page: London.

Hyrkas, K. (1997) "Can Action Research be Applied in Developing Clinical Teaching?" *Journal of Advanced Nursing*, 25, 801–08.

Iles, V. and Sutherland, K. (2001) *Managing Change in the NHS: Organisational Change*. National Coordinating Service for NHS Service Delivery and Organisation. R and D: London.

Kakabadse, A. (1984) "The Politics of a Process Consultant" in A. Kakabadse and C. Parker (eds) *Power, Politics and Organisations*. Wiley: Chicester, 169–83.

Kanter, R.M. (1983) *The Change Masters*. Simon and Schuster: New York.

Kaplan, R. and Norton, D. (1996) *The Balanced Scorecard*. Harvard Business School Press: Boston.

Katz, R. and Kahn, D. (1978) *The Social Psychology of Organisations*. Wiley: New York.

Kelly, D. and Simpson, S. (2001) "Action Research in Action: Reflections on a Project to Introduce Clinical Practice Facilitators to an Acute Hospital Setting." *Journal of Advanced Nursing*, 33, 652–59.

Kelman, H.C. (1969) "Processes of Opinion Change" in W. Bennis, K. Benne and R. Chin, *The Planning of Change*, 2nd ed. Holt, Rinehart and Winston: New York, 222–30

Kieran, D. (1998) "The Role of Culture in the Relationship between the Statutory and Voluntary Sectors in the Provision of Services to the Intellectually Disabled." Unpublished M.Sc. Thesis. University of Dublin: Dublin.

Kilgour, C. and Fleming, V. (2000) "An Action Research Inquiry into a Health Visitor Programme for Parents of Pre-school Children with Behavioural Problems." *Journal of Advanced Nursing*, 32, 682–88.

Kimberly, J.R. and Evanisko, M.J. (1981) "Organisational Innovation: The Influence of Individual, Organisational and Contextual Factors on Hospital Adoption of Technological and Administrative Innovations." *Academy of Management Journal*, 24, 689–713.

King, N. and Anderson, N. (1995) *Innovation and Change in Organisations*. Routledge: London.

Kitzinger, J. (1995) "Introducing Focus Groups." *British Medical Journal*, 311, 299–302.

Kitzinger, J. (1996) "Introducing Focus Groups" in N. Mays and C. Pope (eds) *Qualitative Research in Health Care*, British Medical Journal Publishing Group: London, 36–45.

Klein, D. (1969) "Some Notes on the Dynamics of Resistance to Change: The 'Defender' Role" in W. Bennis, K. Benne and R. Chin, *The Planning of Change*, 2nd ed. Holt, Rinehart and Winston: New York, 498–506.

Kolb, D. (1984) *Experiential Learning*. Prentice-Hall: Upper Saddle River, NJ.

Korman, A.K. (1966) "'Consideration', 'Initiating Structure' and 'Organisational Criteria' – A Review." *Personnel Psychology*, 19, 349–61.

Kotter, J. (1995) "Leading Change: Why Transformation Efforts Fail." *Harvard Business Review*, March–April, 59–67.

Kotter, J. (1996) *Leading Change*. Harvard Business School Press: Boston.

Kotter, J. and Schlesinger, L. (1979) "Choosing Strategies for Change." *Harvard Business Review*, March–April, 106–14.

Lauri, S. and Sainio, C. (1998) "Developing the Nursing Care of Breast Cancer Patients: An Action Research Approach." *Journal of Clinical Nursing*, 7, 424–32.

Legge, K. (1985) *Evaluating Planned Organisational Change*. Academic Press: London.

Lewin, K. (1948) "Group Decision and Social Change." Reproduced in M. Gold (ed.) *The Complete Social Scientist: A Kurt Lewin Reader*. American Psychological Association: Washington, 1997, 265–84.

Likert, R. (1967) *The Human Organisation*. McGraw-Hill: New York.

Lippitt, G. and Lippitt, R. (1978) *The Consulting Process in Action*. Pfeiffer: San Francisco.

MacLachlan, M. and Mc Auliffe, E. (1992) "Overcoming Clinicians' Resistance to Consumer Satisfaction Surveys." *Journal of Management in Medicine*, 6 (3), 52–6.

MacLachlan, M. and Mc Auliffe, E. (1993) "Critical Incidents for Psychology Students in a Refugee Camp: Implications for Counselling." *Counselling Psychology Quarterly*, 6 (1), 3–11.

MacLachlan, M. and Mc Auliffe, E. (2003) "Poverty and Process Skills" in S.C. Carr and T. Sloan (eds) *Poverty and Psychology: Critical Emergent Perspectives*. Kluwer/Plenum: Boston, 226–42.

Mann, F.C. (1957) "Studying and Creating Change: A Means to Understanding Social Organisation." Cited in Burke (2002: 29).

Margulies, N. and Adams, J.D. (1982) *Organisation Development in Health Care Organisations*. Addison-Wesley: Reading, MA.

Marquardt, M. (1999) *Action Learning in Action*. Davies-Black: Palo Alto, CA.

Marsick, V. and Watkins, K. (1999) *Facilitating Learning Organisations*. Gower: Aldershot.

Mc Auliffe, E. (1996) "AIDS: The Barriers to Behaviour Change" in H. Grad, A. Blanco and J. Georgas (eds) *Key Issues in Cross-Cultural Psychology*. Swets and Zeitlinger: Lisse, The Netherlands, 371–86.

Mc Auliffe, E. (1998) "Consumer Involvement in Healthcare" in E. Mc Auliffe and L. Joyce (eds) *A Healthier Future? Managing Healthcare in Ireland*. Institute of Public Administration: Dublin, 286–305.

Mc Auliffe, E., Coghlan, D. and Pathe, A. (2002) "Organisation Development and Change Management in the Irish Health Boards: Current Policies and Practices." *Administration*, 50 (3), 42–63.

Mc Auliffe, E. and MacLachlan M. (1992) "Clinicians' Resistance to Consumer Satisfaction Surveys: What They Never Tell You." *Journal of Management in Medicine*, 6 (3), 47–51.

Mc Auliffe, E. and Ntata, P. (1994) *Youth and AIDS: Baseline Survey of Knowledge Attitudes, and Practices*, UNICEF: Geneva.

McCarthy, G. (1998) "Leadership: Making the Best Use of the Nursing Resource" in E. Mc Auliffe and L. Joyce (eds) *A Healthier Future? Managing Healthcare in Ireland*. Institute of Public Administration: Dublin, 237–56.

McCaughan, N. and Palmer B. (1994) *Systems Thinking for Harassed Managers*. Karnac: London.

McCaugherty, D. (1991) "The Theory-Practice Gap in Nurse Education: Its Causes and Possible Solutions. Findings from an Action Research Study", *Journal of Advanced Nursing*, 16, 1055–61.

McElroy, A., Corben, V. and McLeish, K. (1995) "Developing Care Plan Documentation: An Action Research Project." *Journal of Advanced Nursing*, 3, 193–99.

McGill I. and Beaty, L. (1995) *Action Learning*, 2nd ed. Kogan Page: London.

McGregor, D. (1960) *The Human Side of Enterprise*. McGraw-Hill: New York.

McIlduff, E. and Coghlan, D. (2000) "Understanding and Contending with Passive-Aggressive Behaviour in Teams and Organisations." *Journal of Managerial Psychology*, 15 (7), 716–36.

McKee, R. and Carlson, B. (1999) *The Power to Change*. Grid International Inc: Austin, Tx.

Meehan, C. (2001) "Managers as Healing Agents in Organisations: An Action Research Approach." Unpublished Masters Thesis. University of Dublin: Dublin.

Merry, U. and Brown, G. (1987) *The Neurotic Behavior of Organisations*, Gestalt Institute of Cleveland Press: Cleveland, OH.

Meyer, M.C. (1977) "Six Stages of Demotivation." *International Management*, April, 14–17.

Mintzberg, H. (1997) "Towards Healthier Hospitals." *Health Care Management Review*, 22 (4), 9–18.

Mintzberg, H. (1998) "Covert Leadership: Notes on Managing Professionals." *Harvard Business Review*, November–December, 140–47.

Mohr, L.B. (1969) "Determinants of Innovation in Organisations." *American Political Science Review*, 63, 111–26.

Morgan, G. (1997) *Images of Organisation*. Sage: London.

Morrison B. and Lilford, R. (2001) "How Can Action Research Apply to Health Services?" *Qualitative Health Research*, 11 (4), 436–49.

Morton-Cooper, A. (2000) *Action Research in Health Care*. Blackwell: Oxford.

Nadler, D. (1977) *Feedback and Organisation Development*. Addison-Wesley: Reading, MA.

Nadler, D. (1998) *Champions of Change*. Jossey-Bass: San Francisco.

Neilsen, E.H. (1984) *Becoming an OD Practitioner*. Prentice-Hall: Upper Saddle River, NJ.

Neumann J. (1989) "Why People Don't Participate in Organisational Change" in R. Woodman and W. Pasmore (eds) *Research in Organisational Change and Development*, 3, JAI Press: Greenwich, CT, 181–212.

Nevis, E.C. (1987) *Organisational Consulting: A Gestalt Approach*. Gestalt Institute of Cleveland Press: Cleveland, OH.

Northouse, P. (1997) *Leadership: Theory and Practice*. Sage: London.

Nursing Education Forum (2000) *A Strategy for a Pre-Registration Nursing Education Degree Programme*. Stationary Office: Dublin.

Ochieng, B. (1999) "Use of Reflective Practice in Introducing Change in Management of Pain in a Paediatric Setting." *Journal of Nursing Management*, 7, 113–18.

Office for Health Management (2001) *Clinicians in Management, Discussion Paper 3*. Office For Health Management: Dublin.

Ong, B.N (1993) *The Practice of Health Services Research*. Chapman and Hall: London.

Ong, W.J. (1982) *Orality and Literacy*. Methuen: London.

Ovretveit, J. (1993) *Co-ordinating Community Care: Multidisciplinary Teams and Care Management*. Open University Press: Buckingham.

Owen, H. (1997) *Open Space Technology*. Berrett-Koehler: San Francisco.

Owen, J.M. (1993) *Program Evaluation: Forms and Approaches.* Allen and Unwin: Sydney.

Owen, J.M. and Lambert, F. (1995) "Roles for Evaluation in Learning Organisations." *Evaluation,* 1 (2), 237–50.

Page, S. and Meerabeau, L. (2000) "Achieving Change through Reflective Practice: Closing the Loop." *Nurse Education Today,* 20, 365–72.

Pascale, R., Milleman, M. and Gioja, L. (2000) *Surfing on the Edge of Chaos.* Crown Business: New York.

Pedler, M. (1996) *Action Learning for Managers.* Lemos and Crane: London.

Peters, T.J. and Waterman, R.H. (1982) *In Search of Excellence.* Harper and Row: New York.

Pettigrew, A. (1985) "Towards a Political Theory of Organisational Interventions." *Human Relations,* 28, 191–208.

Pettigrew, A. (ed.) (1987) *The Management of Strategic Change.* Blackwell: Oxford.

Pettigrew, A., Ferlie, E. and McKee, L. (1992) *Shaping Strategic Change.* Sage: London.

Plochg, T. and Klazinga, N.S. (2002) "Community-based Integrated Care: Myth or Must?" *International Journal for Quality in Health Care,* 14 (2), 91–101.

Potter, C., Morgan, P. and Thompson, A. (1994) "Continuous Quality Improvement in an Acute Hospital", *International Journal of Health Care Quality Assurance,* 7 (1), 4–29.

Prather, S., Blake, R. and Mouton, J. (1990) *Behavioral Types and the Art of Patient Management.* PMICS: Los Angeles.

Pratt, J., Gordon, P. and Plamping, D. (1999) *Working Whole Systems.* King's Fund: London.

Preskill, H. and Torres, R. (1999) *Evaluative Inquiry for Learning in Organisations.* Sage: Thousand Oaks, CA.

Quirke, B. (1996) *Communicating Corporate Change.* McGraw-Hill: New York.

Raelin, J.A (2000) *Work-Based Learning: The New Frontier of Management Development.* Prentice-Hall: Upper Saddle River, NJ.

Ramirez, I.L and Bartunek, J.M. (1989) "The Multiple Realities and Experiences of Internal Organisation Development Consultation in Health Care." *Journal of Organisational Change Management,* 2 (1), 40–57.

Rashford, N.S. and Coghlan, D. (1994) *The Dynamics of Organisational Levels: A Change Framework for Managers and Consultants.* Reading, MA: Addison-Wesley.

Reason, P. (1991) "Power and Conflict in Multidisciplinary Collaboration." *Complementary Medical Research,* 5 (3), 144–50.

Reason, P. (1998) "Co-operative Inquiry as a Discipline of Professional Practice." *Journal of Interprofessional Care,* 12, 419–36.

Reason, P. (2001) "Learning and Change through Action Research" in J. Henry (ed.), *Creative Management*, 2nd ed. Sage: London, 182–94.

Reason, P., Chase H.D., Desser, A., Melhuish, C., Morrison, S., Peters, D., Wallstein, D., Webber, V. and Pietroni, P.C. (1992) "Towards a Clinical Framework for Collaboration between General and Complementary Practitioners: Discussion Paper." *Journal of the Royal Society of Medicine*, 85, 161–64.

Reed, J., Pearson, P., Douglas, B., Swinbourne, S. and Wilding, H. (2002) "Going Home from Hospital: An Appreciative Inquiry Study." *Health and Social Care in the Community*, 10 (1), 36–45.

Revans, R. (1998) *ABC of Action Learning*. Lemos and Crane: London.

Rice, A.K. (1990) "Individual, Group and Inter-group Processes" in E. Trist and H. Murray, *The Social Engagement of Social Science, Volume 1: The Social-Psychological Perspective, A Tavistock Anthology*. University of Pennsylvania Press: Philadelphia, 272–83.

Rimmer, T.C. and Johnson, L.L (1998) *Planned Change Theories for Nursing: Review, Analysis and Applications*. Sage: Thousand Oaks, CA.

Rogers, C.R. (1990) "The Characteristics of the Helping Relationship" in H. Kirschenbaum and V. Henderson (eds) *The Carl Rogers Reader*. Constable: London, 108–26.

Rolfe, G. (1996) "Going to Extremes: Action Research, Grounded Practice and the Theory-Practice Gap in Nursing." *Journal of Advanced Nursing*, 24, 1315–20.

Rothwell, W., Sullivan, R. and McLean, G. (1995) *Practising Organisation Development*. Pfeiffer: San Diego.

Sankaran, S., Dick, B., Passfield, B. and Swepson, P. (2001) *Effective Change Management Using Action Learning and Action Research*. Southern Cross University: Lismore, NSW, Australia.

Schein, E.H. (1978) *Career Dynamics: Matching Individual and Organisational Needs*. Addison-Wesley: Reading, MA.

Schein, E.H. (1980) *Organisational Psychology*, 3rd ed. Prentice-Hall: Englewood Cliffs, N.J.

Schein, E.H. (1987) *The Clinical Perspective in Fieldwork*. Sage: Thousand Oaks, CA.

Schein, E.H. (1993) *Career Survival: Strategic Job and Role Planning*. Pfeiffer: San Diego.

Schein, E.H. (1997) "Organisational Learning: What is New?" in M.A. Rahim, R.T. Golembiewski and L.E. Pate (eds) *Current Topics in Management*, Vol. 2. JAI: Greenwich, CT, 11–25.

Schein, E.H. (1999a) *The Corporate Culture Survival Guide*. Jossey-Bass: San Francisco.

Schein, E.H. (1999b) *Process Consultation Revisited: Building the Helping Relationship*. Addison-Wesley: Reading, MA.

Schneider, B. (1991) "Managing Boundaries in Organisations" in M. Kets de Fries and Associates, *Organisations on the Couch: Clinical Perspectives on Organisational Behavior and Change.* Jossey-Bass: San Francisco, 169–70.

Schon, D.A. (1983) *The Reflective Practitioner.* Basic Book: New York.

Schwartz, D. (1984) "Similarities and Differences of Internal and External Consultants" in R.J. Lee and A. Freedman (eds) *Consultation Skills Reading.* NTL Institute: Arlington, VA, 97–100.

Senge, P. (1990) *The Fifth Discipline.* Doubleday: New York.

Senge, P., Roberts, C., Ross, R., Smyth, B. and Kleiner, A. (1994) *The Fifth Discipline Fieldbook.* Nicholas Brealey: London.

Senge, P., Kleiner, A., Roberts, C., Ross, R., Roth, G. and Smyth, B. (1999) *The Dance of Change.* Nicholas Brealey: London.

Senge, P.M. (1997) Communities of Leaders and Learners in Looking Ahead: Implications of the Present, *Harvard Business Review*, September–October, 18–32.

Shani, A.B. and Eberhardt, B. (1987) Parallel Organisation in a Health Care Institution, *Group and Organisation Studies*, 12, 147–73.

Shani, A.B. and Pasmore, W. (1985) "Organisation Inquiry: Towards a New Model of the Action Research Process" in D.D. Warrick (ed.) *Contemporary Organisation Development: Current Thinking and Applications.* Scott Foresman: Glenview, IL, 438–49.

Shepard, H. (1997) "Rules of Thumb for Change Agents" in D. Van Eynde, J. Hoy and D.C Van Eynde (eds) *Organisation Development Classics.* Jossey-Bass: San Francisco, 181–90.

Shirom, A. (1983) "Toward a Theory of Organisation Development Interventions in Unionized Work Settings." *Human Relations* 36 (8), 743–64.

Simons, J. (2002) "An Action Research Study Exploring How Education May Enhance Pain Management in Children." *Nurse Education Today*, 22, 108–17.

Stacey, R. (2001) *Complex Responsive Process in Organisations.* Routledge: London.

Steele, F. (1982) *The Role of the Internal Consultant.* CBI Publishing Company: Boston.

Strasser, S. and Bateman, T.S. (1983) "Perception and Motivation" in S.M. Shortell and A.D. Kaluzny (eds) *Health Care Management.* Wiley: New York, 77–127.

Stufflebeam, D.L. (2000) "The CIPP Model for Evaluation" in D.L. Stufflebeam, G.F. Madaus and T Kellaghan (eds) *Evaluation Models: Viewpoint on Educational and Human Sciences Evaluation,* 2nd ed. Kluwer Academic Publishing Group: Boston, MA, 279–317.

Tannenbaum, R. and Hanna, R. (1985) "Holding On, Letting Go and Moving On: Understanding a Neglected Perspective on Change" in R. Tannenbaum, N. Margulies, F. Massarik et al. *Human Systems Development.* Jossey-Bass: San Francisco, 95–121.

Taylor, B.J. (2000) *Reflective Practice: A Guide for Nurses and Midwives.* Open University Press: Buckingham.

Towell, D. and Harries, C. (1978) *Innovations in Patient Care: An Action Research Study of Change in a Psychiatric Hospital.* Croom Helm: London.

Tremblay, M. (2002) "Curing the Health System by Democratic Dialogue." [French] *Infirmiere du Quebec*, 9 (6), 44–5.

Ury, W. (1991) *Getting Past No.* Business Books: London.

Waclawski, J. and Church, A.C. (2002) *Organisation Development: A Data-Driven Approach to Organisational Change.* Jossey-Bass: San Francisco.

Ward, M. (1994) *Why Your Corporate Culture Change Isn't Working and What to Do about It.* Gower: Aldershot.

Waterman, H., Tillen, D., Dickson, R. and de Koning, K. (2001) "Action Research: A Systematic Review and Guidance for Assessment." *Health Technology Assessment*, 5, 23.

Watkins, J.M. and Mohr, B.J. (2001) *Appreciative Inquiry: Change at the Speed of Imagination.* Jossey-Bass/Pfeiffer: San Francisco.

Watkins, K. and Golembiewski, R.T. (2000). "Rethinking Organisation Development for the Learning Organisation" in R.T Golembiewski (ed.) *Handbook of Organisational Consultation*, 2nd ed. Marcel Dekker: New York, 997–1007.

Watkins, K. and Marsick, V. (1993) *Sculpting the Learning Organisation: Lessons in the Art of Systemic Change.* Jossey-Bass: San Francisco.

Watson, G. (1969) "Resistance to Change" in W. Bennis, K. Benne and R. Chin, *The Planning of Change*, 2nd ed. Holt, Rinehart and Winston: New York, 488–97.

Webb, C. (1989) "Action Research: Philosophy, Methods and Personal Experience." *Journal of Advanced, Nursing*, 14, 403–10.

Webb, C. and Pontin, D. (1997) "Evaluating the Introduction of Primary Nursing: The Use of a Care Plan Audit." *Journal of Clinical Nursing*, 6, 395–401.

Weick, K. and Quinn, R. (1999) "Organisational Change and Development." *Annual Review of Psychology*, 50, 361–86.

Weisbord, M. (1987) *Productive Workplaces.* Jossey-Bass: San Francisco.

Weisbord, M. (1988) "Towards a New Practice of OD: Notes on Snapshooting and Moviemaking" in W.A. Pasmore and R. Woodman (eds) *Research in Organisational Change and Development*, 2. JAI: Greenwich, CT, 59–96.

Weisbord, M. and Janoff, S. (1995) *Future Search.* Berrett-Kohler: San Francisco.

Wheatley, M. (1999) *Leadership and the New Science.* Berrett-Kohler: San Francisco.

Wheelan, S.A. (1999) *Creating Effective Teams.* Sage: Thousand Oaks, CA.

White, D.B. (1999) "The Key to OD in HSOs: Service Quality." *Organisation Development Journal*, 17 (1), 95–102.

White, L.P. and Wooten, K.C. (1986) *Professional Ethics and Practice in Organisation Development*. Praeger: New York.

Winter, R. and Munn-Giddings, C. (2001) *A Handbook for Action Research in Health and Social Care*. Routledge: London.

Worren, N., Ruddle, K. and Moore, K. (1999) "From Organisation Development to Change Management: The Emergence of a New Profession." *Journal of Applied Behavioral Science*, 35, 273–86.

Zaleznik, A. (1977) "Managers and Leaders: Are They Different?" *Harvard Business Review*, 55 (3), 67–78.

Zaltman, G. and, Duncan, R. (1977) *Strategies for Planned Change*. Wiley: New York.

Indices

SUBJECT INDEX